CBD OIL

Everyday Secrets

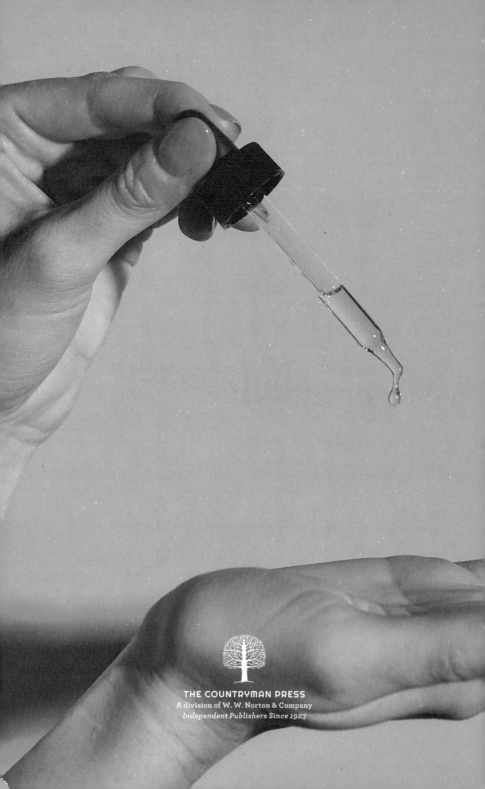

THE COUNTRYMAN PRESS
A division of W. W. Norton & Company
Independent Publishers Since 1923

A LIFESTYLE GUIDE TO HEMP-DERIVED HEALTH AND WELLNESS

CBD

Everyday Secrets

OIL

GRETCHEN LIDICKER

FOREWORD BY TIFFANY LESTER, MD

DISCLAIMER: This volume is intended as a general information resource. It is not a substitute for, and should not be deemed to include, legal or medical advice.

CBD oil can have or cause significant physical effects. If you have been diagnosed with, or suspect you may have, any medical or psychological condition, or if you are pregnant or considering pregnancy, consult your doctor or other professional healthcare provider before using CBD oil. Do not give CBD to children or the elderly except on the advice of a physician.

References in this book to third-party organizations, tools, products, and services are for general information purposes only. Neither the publisher nor the author can guarantee that any particular practice or resource will be useful or appropriate to the reader. Web addresses included in this book reflect links existing as of the date of first publication. The publisher is not responsible for the content of any website, blog, or information page other than its own.

For information about permission to reproduce selections from this book, write to Permissions, The Countryman Press, 500 Fifth Avenue, New York, NY 10110

For information about special discounts for bulk purchases, please contact W. W. Norton Special Sales at specialsales@wwnorton.com or 800-233-4830

Manufacturing by Versa Press
Book design by Tiani Kennedy
Production manager: Devon Zahn

The Countryman Press
www.countrymanpress.com

A division of W. W. Norton & Company, Inc
500 Fifth Avenue, New York, NY 10110
www.wwnorton.com

978-1-68268-340-8 (pbk.)

10 9 8 7 6 5 4 3 2 1

To my parents,
who never acted like any of my dreams were
too big or too crazy. Thanks for always,
always, always having my back.

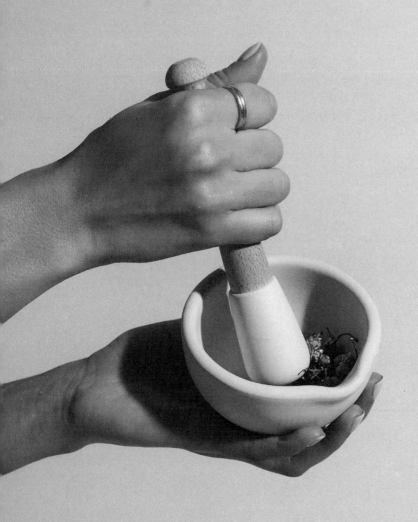

CONTENTS

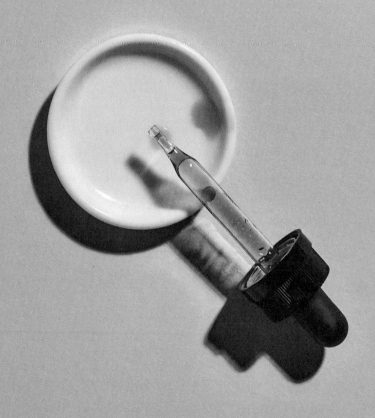

FOREWORD

This book—*CBD Oil: Everyday Secrets*—is what I wish had been available when I first started to delve into the world of CBD. I moved to San Francisco in October 2016 to become medical director at Parsley Health. As a doctor, I had only heard of the use of Marinol (a synthetic cannabinoid compound) for treating refractory nausea and AIDS-associated weight loss. And as a human, I had never even smoked weed, and honestly, I was slightly judgmental of people who did! I am the last person my friends and family would expect to try CBD or THC in any form or fashion.

Now fast-forward eighteen months. I live in a state where marijuana is legal for both medical and recreational use as of January 1, 2018. My patients ask my opinion about the reported health benefits of CBD on a weekly basis for conditions ranging from insomnia to anxiety to menstrual cramps.

I quickly realized that I needed to educate myself about this herb and the medicinal benefits. As an advocate of functional medicine that looks at the root cause of disease, I was excited to learn about this potential treatment. But even though I take a more holistic approach to healthcare, there can still be a stigma when it comes to discussing CBD with your doctor.

Currently there isn't an abundance of research in the United States to learn about how the endocannabinoid system works to treat pain and lessen anxiety—which is why a book like this is essential to start the necessary conversation about the benefits of CBD. I first met Gretchen last year at the annual mindbodygreen revitalize conference in Arizona. As a longtime writer for mbg, I loved meeting all the amazing editors in person. In this book, Gretchen takes you on a journey of the basics of CBD, why it's useful, the whole CBD-to-THC ratio situation, and even delicious recipes to start experimenting in your own kitchen.

My own bias against CBD came from the strict laws that were in place when I was growing up as an '80s baby in the Midwest, adopting my parents' views around marijuana and seeing members of my community jailed for illegal possession. I was a rule follower, not a rule breaker, and I knew that my dream of becoming a doctor didn't exactly go hand in hand with having a criminal record. Living in California has allowed me to legally experiment with the variations of CBD, including teas, balms, bath salts, edibles, and tinctures. This has led me to be more comfortable having the conversation with patients about the myriad of treatment options. Having physicians who are open to a dialogue about this natural remedy is important for truly comprehensive health care.

CBD Oil: Everyday Secrets gives newcomers a great foundation, and even self-proclaimed CBD experts will gain knowledge from this book. Enjoy!

Tiffany Lester, MD
Medical Director, Parsley Health
San Francisco
2018

INTRODUCTION

Meet CBD, Nature's Greatest Plant Medicine

It's likely you've been hearing some chatter about CBD oil lately, either on the Internet, in a magazine, as a featured ingredient at your local juice bar, or on your favorite wellness guru's Instagram page. You probably wondered: *What's that?* With a quick Google search, you learned that CBD is actually a compound derived from the hemp plant, and you thought to yourself: *Hmm, that's interesting.* With a little bit more research, it's likely that you uncovered a few wellness experts singing its praises as an all-natural remedy for anxiety or chronic inflammation: *That sounds pretty great.*

If you really got into it, you uncovered some articles that pose CBD as a possible tool in fighting the opioid epidemic, or read how it's been life-changing for children with rare seizure disorders, or how it could potentially help with depression, schizophrenia, acne, irritable bowel syndrome . . . I think you get the point. You said out loud this time: "It can't possibly do all that, can it?" The many, many (many) claims about the healing properties and potential of CBD make it seem pretty amazing—and pretty hard to believe.

The notion of an all-natural plant compound that works in such a variety of ways is appealing, but it also sets off some major red flags. If you decided to dive a little deeper into the science of CBD, you'd quickly realize that the topic isn't a simple one. Forget the actual science—even questions as basic as "Where do I buy CBD?" "What's it made from?" or "Is it legal?" can be difficult to answer. Sadly, the more you scroll through your search page results, the more confused you become; it can seem like there's more conflicting information out there than actual facts. More red flags!

Believe me, I get it. When I first started researching CBD, I was shocked at the lack of clear, factual information out there, even when it came to basic information like how much CBD a person should take. You'd think that, at least, would be pretty black-and-white. (Spoiler alert: It's not!) This lack of information exists for a *lot* of reasons—many of which we'll cover throughout the course of this book—but for now, let's just admit that it makes CBD feel a little too mysterious, at least for most of us.

Luckily, though, you sought out—or stumbled upon—this book, which was written to solve exactly that problem. Together, we'll go through important things to know about CBD, from the basics of its pharmacology to its healing benefits to some guidelines on dosage and safety. I'll talk about how to use CBD and where to buy it and why some CBD companies are better than others. Finally and most importantly, we'll have some fun. By bringing CBD into the kitchen and learning how to incorporate it into beauty and self-care routines, you can really take advantage of its healing benefits. Because that's the whole point, right?

If you're skeptical about CBD, that is totally understandable. In fact, I applaud you, and I want to thank you for picking up this book. (Because skepticism alone doesn't get us anywhere unless we also toss in a little open-mindedness.) Maybe you're suspicious of all the CBD hype and its seemingly endless healing properties, or maybe you're just not sure about inviting a compound with such a close relationship to marijuana into your home. Whatever the reason, the first step is to learn more.

And that's where I come in. If you're wondering about me, it's understandable, and believe me, I don't take it personally. It can be hard to find information about CBD written by someone who isn't also trying to sell it to you. How can you trust me? Because I'm writing this book as a CBD industry outsider, and in many ways I'm learning right alongside you. That being said, as the health editor at mindbodygreen—a major health and wellness media company that covers everything from gut health and food allergies to environmental toxins and mindful parenting—I'm a wellness industry insider, and I've been working on the clinical and academic side of integrative and functional medicine for years. This means I've spent a lot of time swimming through wellness trends, trying to separate fact from fiction; fad from fundamental pillar of health; scientific proof from manipulation of data. I'm writing this book as someone who's simply trying to learn more about CBD and present its case to all of you. And then let you decide for yourself.

In my experience, the best way to start this journey is with the cold, hard facts. Are you ready? Remember, we're in this together.

10 Things Everyone Gets Wrong About CBD

Because of its close relationship with marijuana, there's a lot of stigma surrounding cannabidiol, abbreviated as CBD. But as with many stigmas, like those related to mental health issues or addiction, CBD's stigma stems from misinformation or a lack of knowledge about the real complexities of an issue. Sadly, trying to educate yourself on CBD can leave you totally confused and reading a lot of conflicting information. For example, one website will claim that CBD is the ultimate insomnia cure, while another says that it's an all-natural energy stimulant that can keep you up at night. One article will tell you that CBD is absorbed through the skin, and the next will say that can't possibly be true. These different pieces of information are hard to put together into one cohesive understanding—or even any kind of understanding at all.

Sometimes when a topic is complex or overwhelming, it's easier to start with what you know is wrong before you turn to facts that you think might be true. It's kind of like changing careers: Making a list of jobs you know you don't want feels a lot less daunting than making a list of those you do. With that in mind, here are ten major misconceptions about CBD.

1. **CBD is made from hemp.** We're really starting out with a bang! But this one is absolutely critical. CBD is one of the many chemical compounds present in the *Cannabis sativa* plant, which includes both marijuana and hemp. These compounds are often referred to as *phytocannabinoids*. *Phyto* tells us that they come from a plant and *cannabinoid* is the name given to a group of closely related compounds found both inside and outside the body. We'll do a deep dive into the difference between hemp and marijuana, but for now, just remember that they are both cannabis, and CBD can be derived from either.

2. **CBD is THC without the high.** Historically (and when we were in high school), the only cannabinoid people really cared about was THC—which is responsible for the mind-altering effects of marijuana. But as CBD quickly gains recognition in both the medical and wellness communities, it's easy to assume that the only difference between THC and CBD has to do with intoxication. That's entirely untrue. Because though they are both from the same plant, they are two completely distinct compounds that interact *very differently* in the body. CBD is considered nonintoxicating, but we fail to recognize its unique nature when we assume it's just THC without the high.

3. **CBD is nonpsychoactive.** So now that we've gotten number two out of the way, let's get more specific about how CBD actually affects the body and the brain. To be clear: *CBD will not get you stoned.* But it does have some sort of effect on the brain, and therefore the word I and a lot of other CBD experts prefer to use when describing it is *nonintoxicating*. Psychoactive means "affecting the mind or behavior," and because CBD has known effects on the brain and is used as a treatment for anxiety, PTSD, seizure disorders, and depression (and the list goes on), by nature it can't really be described as "nonpsychoactive."

4. **CBD is legal in all fifty states.** If I had a penny for every time I read or heard someone say that CBD was legal in all fifty states! In fact, I've frequently heard this from people who sell CBD. Now, to resist opening a massive can of worms and asking you to read all of chapter 3 (where I talk about the legal status of CBD in detail) right now, let's just leave it at this: Under federal law, CBD is classified as a Schedule 1 substance because it's derived from *Cannabis sativa*, which falls under the same class. That being said, various laws have been passed that allow CBD to be extracted and then manufactured, sold, studied, and taken as long as some specific requirements are met. More on this later, I promise.

5. **CBD is only for crunchy granola people.** A lot of people think CBD is only for "alternative" people who also lather themselves in Aztec clay and brew their own kombucha. And while there is absolutely nothing wrong with Aztec clay, CBD was actually first described by an Israeli scientist in a white lab coat and was made famous in the United States by a five-year-old girl named Charlotte. Some of the biggest movers and shakers in the CBD industry have been parents and scientists and teachers, many of whom admitted they were against the legalization of cannabis until they discovered CBD. It has also caused quite a few high-profile doctors—including Dr. Sanjay Gupta, a famous neurosurgeon and Emmy Award–winning medical reporter—to completely change their tune on cannabis. That being said, the crunchy granola wellness industry people have definitely welcomed CBD with open arms, and for good reason.
   Oh, and there's nothing wrong with kombucha, either.

6. **CBD is a recent discovery.** Because of all the buzz CBD has been getting lately, it's easy to assume it's a recent discovery that will change the face of medicine in a whirlwind of new studies and information. Well, to make a long story short, we've known about CBD— and even some of its specific healing benefits like its anti-seizure

properties—for decades. That being said, the hemp-based CBD products we're seeing on the market now are definitely a newer phenomenon, and they really seem to be making waves. So though we didn't just discover it, I do think we're entering a new era for CBD.

7. **CBD is from hemp and THC is from marijuana.** Out of all the myths about CBD, this one might be the most popular. In fact, I once believed it myself (that's just between us). But to say that hemp contains only CBD and marijuana contains only THC is a massive oversimplification of both the difference between hemp and marijuana and the way these compounds appear in the plants. This is true for many reasons, but for now let's just think about it like this: There are a *ton* of different types of cannabis, and each has a different ratio of CBD to THC. This ratio can vary between strains, and even between individual plants—and just because a plant is low in THC doesn't mean it will automatically be high in CBD. Historically, marijuana has been bred to be higher in THC because the goal was always to use it for recreation, but things are really changing here, and the lines are getting majorly blurred.

8. **When you buy CBD, you have no idea what you are really getting.** Because CBD occupies a legal gray area, it's hard to know exactly how the quality of CBD supplements is being overseen. I won't sugarcoat it: when you buy CBD products, you're putting a *lot* of trust in the hands of the person who is manufacturing your CBD, as with any supplements or vitamins. That being said, many CBD companies are using third-party testing to show consumers that they adhere to the highest standards of quality and manufacturing, which is why chapter 8, on finding good CBD products, is the most important chapter in this book. The take-home message? There is a way to take CBD and feel secure that what's on the label is actually what's in the bottle.

9. **CBD has barely been studied, and we don't know how it works.** A lot of people say that we don't know anything about CBD. To this I would say yes, there's a lot we don't know, but we do know quite a bit about CBD's safety profile and its mechanism of action in the body. In large part, this is due to the fact that there are CBD-based pharmaceutical drugs approved for use in places like Europe and Canada (and one was approved by the Food and Drug Administration in the United States in 2018). This means that we know quite a bit about how it interacts with the body, and different doses and preparations of CBD have been studied extensively for safety and efficacy in human clinical trials.

10. **CBD is good and THC is bad.** Once you start learning more about CBD, it's easy to start believing that CBD is everything good about cannabis and therefore THC embodies all the negative aspects. It is true that THC represents the more recreational side of the plant (and also has more negative side effects associated with it), but THC has incredible healing benefits, on its own and especially when combined with CBD and other cannabinoids.

You might be feeling a little shell-shocked. That was a lot at once! It seems like there are so many misconceptions when it comes to CBD. So is *anything* an undisputed fact? As I mentioned before, researchers have actually uncovered quite a bit about the science of CBD, so that's where we'll begin.

The Science of CBD

If you're a science nerd like me, then congratulations! This will be your favorite chapter. If you hate science and still have nightmares about high school chemistry, then hang tight and trust me, this will be more fun than you think.

CANNABINOIDS AND THE ENDOCANNABINOID SYSTEM

As we learned before, CBD and THC are both cannabinoids, but they are far from the only ones! *Cannabinoid* is a name given to a big group of chemically similar compounds. There are phytocannabinoids (these come from plants and include CBD and THC) and endocannabinoids (these are naturally produced inside the body) and even synthetic cannabinoids (which are created in a lab). And while THC and CBD are the most well-known, there are actually more than eighty different cannabinoids and as many as four hundred different chemical compounds inside the cannabis plant. The endocannabinoids in your body—and the phytocannabinoids or synthetic cannabinoids that you ingest—interact with a larger entity within the body called the endocannabinoid system (ECS).

GETTING TO KNOW THE ENDOCANNABINOID SYSTEM

The ECS is a major system in the body (sort of like the hormone systems you may have learned about in health class) and mostly consists of endocannabinoids, their receptors, and a variety of regulatory and metabolic enzymes that play a part in the detailed workings of the system. Cannabinoid receptors are present all over the body in tissues like the brain, gastrointestinal tract, reproductive system, spleen, arteries, and even the heart. Some like to refer to the ECS as the "master regulatory system" because it seems to be everywhere and do everything. When you learn this, it starts to make more sense that CBD also seems to "do it all."

The main job of the ECS is to maintain homeostasis (i.e., help the body regulate itself regardless of what's going on around it), and it's also considered an adaptogenic system, which means it plays a role in how our bodies respond to things like pain, anxiety, and stress. You'll sometimes hear CBD referred to as an *adaptogen*, and this is why. The ECS plays a big role in inflammation and communicates directly with important parts of the body like the central nervous system and the gastrointestinal tract. Many experts think that the ECS is involved, at least to some extent, in almost all disease and dysfunction, which we'll delve deeper into in chapter 5.

UNDERSTANDING ENDOCANNABINOID TONE

The close relationship between the ECS and overall health led scientists to develop the term *endocannabinoid tone*, which refers to the general health status of one's endocannabinoid system. When one has a low endocannabinoid tone, one is essentially deficient in endocannabinoids, a condition that has been linked to disorders like chronic pain, fibromyalgia, glaucoma, and irritable bowel syndrome. One study conducted in Italy actually showed that people with chronic migraine diagnoses had lower concentrations of endocannabinoids in their bodies. This newfound knowledge has prompted researchers to coin the term "clinical endocannabinoid deficiency."

One's individual endocannabinoid tone has a lot to do with various lifestyle factors like how healthy one's gut microbiome is and how much one exercises. This is really no surprise, given that the ECS talks to just about every organ in the body, but it does make for a new, interesting way to measure people's overall health through their endocannabinoid tone.

GETTING ACQUAINTED WITH YOUR BODY'S NATURAL CANNABINOIDS

We know that CBD and THC are two common phytocannabinoids, but what do the cannabinoids inside our bodies (remember, these are called *endocannabinoids*) look like, and what do they do? The two endocannabinoids that we know the most about are anandamide (AEA), which is also known as the "bliss molecule," and 2-Arachidonoylglycerol (2-AG). These chemicals are abundant in the brain, are synthesized from fatty acids in the body on demand, and are known to play a role in everything from appetite and depression to fertility and pain management.

So what do AEA and 2-AG actually do on a larger scale? In his book *Smoke Signals*, Martin Lee explained that endocannabinoids function as subtle sensing devices, and when they are activated, they put the brakes on excessive activity of the body's many systems. As he put it: "Endocannabinoids are the only neurotransmitters known to engage in 'retrograde signaling,' a unique form of intracellular communication that inhibits immune response, reduces inflammation, relaxes musculature, lowers blood pressure, dilates bronchial passages, . . . and normalizes overstimulated nerves." In other words, they tell your body to chill the hell out, which is exactly what most of our bodies (and brains) need to hear.

If you're wondering how researchers discovered all this, you have impeccable timing, because I'm about to tell you! Interestingly, the endocannabinoid system and endocannabinoids were discovered as a result of studying phytocannabinoids in cannabis. Essentially, once scientists figured out which receptors THC and CBD were reacting with in the body, they learned that there were cannabinoids already being made by the body that were interacting with those same receptors. With that knowledge, they were then able to describe the whole endocannabinoid system in all its glory.

This seems a little backward, but there are actually quite a few instances in history when studying plants led to the discovery of an entire bodily system. One good example is when scientists were studying the receptor sites for opium, the plant that opioid narcotic pain-killers are based on. They discovered that those same receptor sites interact with natural chemicals in the body called *endorphins*. Endorphins are often described as "feel-good chemicals" and are produced by the brain when we're in pain or under high amounts of stress. Basically, endorphins are the body's natural opiates, and AEA and 2-AG are the body's natural cannabinoids.

HOW CBD WORKS IN THE BODY AND BRAIN

As we already know, cannabinoids affect us because they interact with receptors on our cells, many of which are called *cannabinoid receptors*. These receptors are found all over our bodies, and researchers have identified two specific types of cannabinoid receptors, called CB_1 and CB_2.

In general, CB_1 receptors are found mostly in the brain and the central nervous system, and CB_2 receptors are closely tied to the activity of the immune system. THC interacts strongly with both CB_1 and CB_2 receptors, meaning it binds with the receptor and elicits a response. An easy way to think about this is that THC is a key and the receptors are a lock. When the lock and key match, the door is opened. THC's activation of CB_1 receptors is responsible for the altered state of mind we experience from smoking marijuana, so you won't be surprised when I tell you that CBD does not have a strong affinity for CB_1 receptors (meaning it's not the right key for the lock). You might be surprised, however, to learn that CBD doesn't directly activate CB_2 receptors, either. Instead, CBD interacts with the body through a bunch of other mechanisms—some of which indirectly influence the activity of CB_1 and CB_2 receptors, but not in a lock-and-key sort of way.

For a long time it was thought that all cannabinoids reacted with the body through CB_1 and CB_2, but now we know that instead, CBD reacts with several other noncannabinoid receptors and ion channels. This can quickly get complicated, and there's still a lot to learn about

A Short Introduction to Cannabinoids

Out of all the dozens of cannabinoids in the cannabis plant, THC and CBD are the most abundant. This fact, and the knowledge that THC is the major intoxicating compound in cannabis, have made CBD and THC the most prominent of all the cannabinoids. But as I mentioned earlier, there are at least a hundred different cannabinoids, and as the science of cannabis-based health and wellness develops, we'll be hearing more and more about them. We'll also be hearing a lot more about a phenomenon called the *entourage effect*, where cannabinoids work together to increase each other's overall healing potential. The entourage effect suggests that using the whole plant at once is more powerful than using individual cannabinoids on their own.

Looking at the full gamut of cannabinoids is especially beneficial, because while each one has its own unique healing benefits, each one also has its limitations. THC, for example, is limited by its intoxicating effects and by the simple fact that some people do not tolerate it as well as others. Luckily, a lot of the other cannabinoids have some equally cool healing properties and fewer adverse effects. CBD is the most popular of them, but many of these other phytocannabinoids have barely been studied. Here are some of them and their suspected properties.

- **Cannabigerol (CBG):** antimicrobial, anticancer, anti-inflammatory, antianxiety, antidepressant, reduces blood pressure
- **Cannabinol (CBN):** promotes sleep, relieves pain, stimulates appetite, antimicrobial, antispasmodic
- **Cannabichromene (CBC):** relieves pain, anti-inflammatory, anticancer, antianxiety, antimicrobial
- **Tetrahydrocannabivarin (THCV):** relieves pain, stimulates appetite, anti-seizure, antianxiety
- **Tetrahydrocannabinolic acid (THCA), the nonintoxicating "parent" of THC:** anti-nausea, anti-seizure, anticancer, antispasmodic
- **Cannabidiolic acid (CBDA), the nonintoxicating "parent" of CBD:** anti-nausea, anticancer, anti-inflammatory

Even more interesting, some researchers suspect that cannabinoids may exist in different types of plants, prompting the authors of a 2010 study—titled *Phytocannabinoids beyond the Cannabis plant: Do they exist?* and published in the *British Journal of Pharmacology*—to define phytocannabinoids not just as compounds in the cannabis plant, but as "any plant-derived natural product capable of either directly interacting with cannabinoid receptors or sharing chemical similarity with cannabinoids or both." A few researchers have even claimed that they extracted CBD from the Humulus plant, which is more commonly known as hops and used in beer flavoring.

the myriad ways CBD influences our physiology, so I'll just cover some of the most interesting points and keep moving so the science-fearing among you don't get too impatient with me.

One of the most important ways CBD interacts with our bodies is through G protein-coupled receptors, or *GPCRs*. GPCRs are a big deal—in fact, they're the most common and diverse group of receptors in our bodies. They do a lot, but mainly they sit on the surface of our cells and act like in-boxes, allowing cells to communicate with their surroundings and with each other. Knowing this, you might suspect that they play a major role in medicine, and you'd be right! Scientists think that as much as 50 percent of all medicines bind with these GPCRs to create the desired effect in the body.

When talking about how CBD interacts with our bodies, I'd be remiss if I didn't mention neurotransmitters—the chemicals swimming around in our brains responsible for regulating our mood and behavior—right off the bat. It's likely you've heard of common neurotransmitters like oxytocin and GABA at least once or twice before. If this sparks your interest, I'll talk a lot more about exactly how CBD interacts with these neurotransmitters when I talk about its potential mental health benefits.

CBD also appears to influence the activity of calcium in the body, which is an important mineral for the activity of our muscles and nerves. CBD has also been shown to work as something called an *allosteric modulator*, which means that instead of simply binding to the active site on a receptor like THC does, it can bind to other parts of the receptor and influence its activity that way. I'll get into this more later as well.

If this all sounds really complicated to you, I'm here to assure you that it *is* really complicated. CBD interacts with the body in too many ways to count—or even to put in a book about CBD—so for now, I'll just focus on the fact that CBD acts like a multi-targeted drug, and I'll hit on a lot of its specific activities when I talk about its benefits. There is one characteristic of CBD, however, that I need to talk about now—and that is its ability to act as an antioxidant. CBD's antioxidant activity is why it's such a powerful ingredient to add to beauty and skin-care routines and also explains why it has many of the benefits we talk about in Chapter 5.

THE ANTIOXIDANT POWER OF CBD

Antioxidants are front and center in skin care, and that's because of their antiaging and skin-rejuvenating properties. It's impossible to walk through the ground floor of a department store and not be surrounded by serums, oils, and creams infused with antioxidants. But have you ever thought about what an antioxidant really is? If not, don't worry, because I have—a lot. And now I'm going to tell you everything you need to know.

In short, antioxidants are molecules that help us stay healthy, and they do this by fighting off free radicals. Free radicals are substances produced naturally in the body at low levels, but when we're sick or exposed to toxins (like from too much alcohol, pollution, cigarette smoke, or even too much stress), they can spin out of control and cause damage called *oxidative stress*.

Oxidative stress is bad news for our health and has been linked to premature aging and cellular damage, which spells disease (more specifically, cancer). The science of exactly how antioxidants work to neutralize free radicals and protect the body from cellular damage is fascinating, but if reading up on unpaired electrons and atomic orbitals doesn't sound like your version of fun, just remember that ultimately, antioxidants protect us from cellular damage, and the right balance of antioxidants and free radicals is crucial to living a long and healthy life. Antioxidants are so popular in skin care because everything I just described applies to the life and health of our skin as well.

Lucky for us, our bodies naturally produce a certain amount of antioxidants, and you can also get them from foods like fruits and vegetables, especially colorful ones. Have you ever had someone tell you to eat the rainbow? This is just another way of saying "Eat a wide variety of antioxidants." You've likely heard of common foods—like berries, carrots, red wine, and dark chocolate—praised for their high levels of antioxidants (some common ones are the beta-carotene found in carrots, resveratrol in wine, and flavonoids in chocolate). Substances like algae and the compounds in the cannabis plant are also potent antioxidants, which makes them a great addition to both your diet and skin-care routine.

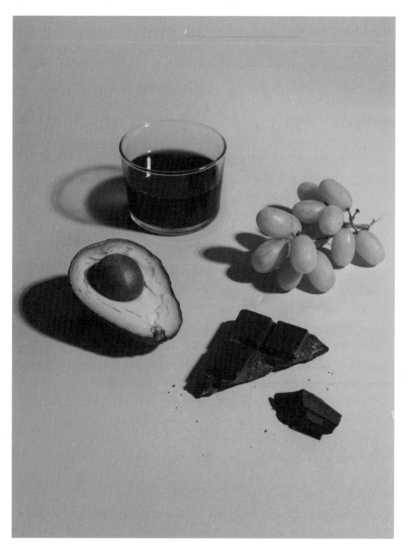

How CBD Changed My Mind About Cannabis

It was late summer, and my then boyfriend and I decided it would be fun to smoke a joint. We jumped in the car, Pitbull playing on the radio, and picked up the "goods" from the parking lot of a local strip mall (do you feel like you're in the moment yet?). We went home and a few minutes after my first puff, I felt like someone was blowing up a balloon in my head. My heart started racing, I felt cold, my brain was firing on all cylinders. I got up to stumble out for some fresh air, and on the way back, I fainted. My then boyfriend (bless him) caught me before I hit the ground, dragged me to the closest piece of furniture, and sat with me for hours convincing me I wasn't having a heart attack until I finally felt like myself again. This was the day that I wrote off the "healing powers" of cannabis.

WHY NEGATIVE REACTIONS TO CANNABIS ARE NEGATIVE REACTIONS TO THC

In telling you this story, I'm doing more than just embarrassing myself and somehow making my ex-boyfriend look like a hero. (Don't you hate when that happens?) I'm trying to make a point, which is that I, like so many other people, have had really negative experiences with cannabis. Due to my violent reactions (yes, sadly, there are a few more stories like the one above), I couldn't enjoy smoking marijuana even if I wanted to. And to be honest, I'd always thought that the healing powers of cannabis were a bit overexaggerated, perpetuated by people who just wanted to get high without fear of arrest. At the very least, I thought that these powers simply didn't apply to me.

And then came CBD oil. When I started learning about this compound, I proceeded with extreme caution. I liked the idea that I could harness the powers of cannabis without the high and the fainting (I'd like to avoid that in the future), but just CBD's connection with the plant that had caused me so much misery made me very nervous. As I learned more about cannabis, however, I realized that my negative reactions to marijuana were likely due to very high-THC strains of the plant. That's what you get when you buy it from the guy at the mall, I suppose.

HOW TO GET THE BENEFITS OF CANNABIS WITHOUT GETTING SUPER STONED

When the federal government made cannabis illegal, it was no longer thought of as a healing plant with medicinal value and people started using it strictly for recreation. During this time, higher-THC strains became dominant. This makes sense when you think about it: Stronger marijuana gets sold for more money. These high-THC strains can still have medicinal value, but they are more likely to cause paranoia, irritation, a racing heart, hallucinations, headaches, and other negative side effects so many experience from smoking marijuana recreationally. It wasn't until relatively recently that anyone even knew what to do with cannabis plants that were naturally high in CBD and low in THC. Luckily, experts are now exploring the whole spectrum of CBD-to-THC ratios, and when I learned this, I started to open up to the idea that I might benefit from some of them.

Begrudgingly, I concluded that if it wasn't cannabis as a whole that was evil and useless, my true enemy must have been THC. It is, after all, the compound with all the downsides, while CBD has virtually none (that we know of so far). But as I went further down the rabbit hole, I realized that it can be difficult to talk about CBD without also talking about THC.

CBD AND THC: A LOVE STORY

Many of you are probably surprised by the amount of time and attention THC has been getting in this book. (It was supposed to be about *CBD oil*, Gretchen!) I hear you, and honestly, I am surprised to be *writing* this much about THC. But I realized that in so many ways—just like your best friend's boyfriend that you're not crazy about but you know she's going to marry—if you care about CBD, you have to care about THC, too.

Earlier I established that CBD and THC work together in the body, so let's talk about exactly what that means. You know that THC is intoxicating, and when you get too much of it, it can cause unpleasant side effects. In stark contrast, multiple studies have referred to CBD having antipsychotic properties and it is even being tested as an adjunctive therapy in schizophrenia. On top of these general antipsychotic properties, CBD works to directly temper the intoxicating effects of THC in the body.

Remember when we talked about how THC activates CB_1 receptors, which cause intoxication? Well, CBD actually works to limit the intoxicating effects of THC by working as an allosteric modulator of CB_1 receptors. This explains the fact that although THC is known for causing anxiety, a racing heart, and even full-blown panic attacks, CBD has been shown to reduce anxiety in general, as well as anxiety induced by too much THC.

Reading this, it can start to feel like CBD is nothing more than the anti-THC. But as described in chapter 1, it's so much more than that. It's important to think of CBD as its own unique compound; THC and CBD are neither opposites nor identical twins. One study, published in the journal *Medical Hypotheses*, put it well by saying that "the combination of THC and CBD increases clinical efficacy while reducing adverse events." In other words, THC and CBD balance each other out and help each other work more effectively at the same time.

So while it pained me to admit it at first, in many ways, CBD and

THC are like the perfect couple. They're opposites in a lot of ways, the same in others; they balance each other out in the most important ways, and they're even better together than they are alone. This really makes you consider the idea that maybe—in small doses—that friend's boyfriend isn't quite as bad as you think.

The History and Politics of Hemp

It comes as a surprise to many, but cannabis has been used for its edible seeds and to make rope, clothing, and paper since Neolithic times. Medicinally, it was used to treat a host of different symptoms and diseases, like gout, malaria, fever, and pain, by doctors, shamans, and druids. One of the oldest known pharmacopoeias (a book that healers used to describe and identify medicinal compounds), called the *Pen-Ts'ao Ching*, contains an entire section on cannabis and how to use it for rheumatic pain, digestive issues, and even conditions like endometriosis.

Cannabis continued to be used as a versatile plant medicine well into the modern era; there's even evidence that Queen Victoria used CBD to treat menstrual cramps in the 1800s, and it was frequently used by Western doctors in the nineteenth century to relieve pain. Cannabis used to be a legitimate medicine, and it was even dispensed at pharmacies in the United States.

Everything changed in the 1930s, when the film *Reefer Madness*, which painted the plant as a corrupting influence, was released, and powerful public figures started denouncing the benefits of the plant.

Cannabis became, and has remained, a social justice issue. Initially, the plant was associated with Mexican immigrants coming to the United States and was used by many to malign their character and create panic. Even today, black Americans are 3.73 times more likely to be arrested for marijuana possession than white Americans. The anticannabis message permeated American culture, and people started referring to cannabis as *marijuana*. Memories of its therapeutic value quickly faded away. Cannabis became more or less illegal with the passing of the Marihuana Tax Act of 1937. In the 1970s, Richard Nixon sounded the alarm and the War on Drugs began; the Controlled Substances Act labeled cannabis (and all its derivatives) a Schedule 1 substance, which means that it has "no known medicinal value."

ISRAEL, PROP 215, AND RESEARCH ON CBD

Since then, cannabis has slowly fought its way back into a positive light and is just now regaining acceptance for its medicinal properties in the United States. In other areas of the world, however, research on cannabis continued to move forward. One country (and one scientist) in particular did a lot of the heavy lifting in the field of cannabis research while the United States was busy jailing people for smoking it. That country was Israel, and the scientist is Dr. Raphael Mechoulam. Both are recognized as world leaders in cannabinoid medicine.

The first cannabinoid to be isolated was cannabinol, or CBN, and this may have happened as early as the late 1800s. The isolation of CBD and THC followed in the 1940s, but it wasn't until the 1960s that the structure of CBD was actually described by Dr. Mechoulam in his lab in Israel. Over the course of his career, Mechoulam has published hundreds of scientific papers on cannabinoids and was also the first to describe THC, the first to synthesize both CBD and THC, and the first to discover how THC interacts with brain receptors. Not surprisingly, he's widely known as the "father of cannabis."

Thanks to Mechoulam and a few other key scientists, there's a lot of great basic research on CBD and other cannabinoids. And these same researchers have also made strides when it comes to learning how cannabinoids can benefit our health. In the 1980s, Mechoulam and researchers from the Hebrew University of Jerusalem and the São Paulo Medicine Faculty of Santa Casa conducted a study testing the effects of 300 milligrams of cannabidiol on eight epileptic patients. After four months, half of these patients had stopped having seizures, and three others saw a decrease in the number of seizures suffered. Sadly, however, the use of CBD to treat epilepsy didn't gain real steam in the years after this study was published, which likely had a lot to do with the stigma against the plant in certain parts of the world.

In 1996, California voters passed Proposition 215, which made it the first state to legalize medical marijuana. And although some research was being conducted at the time, this sparked a new era in which scientists became interested in the medical purposes of cannabis and a more mainstream acceptance of the plant was on the horizon. Keep in mind that at the same time, marijuana was being sold illegally for recreational use all over the country, and high-CBD strains of the plant were largely forgotten, deemed totally unsellable.

Things started to change in the early 2000s when a small pharmaceutical company called GW Pharmaceuticals started developing a CBD-based drug for multiple sclerosis—which is an autoimmune disease characterized by chronic pain—that had a 1:1 ratio of CBD to THC. Slowly but surely, cannabis was being nudged into acceptance.

CHARLOTTE FIGI AND HIGH-CBD CANNABIS

In 2013, things really changed when CNN covered the story of a little girl named Charlotte Figi. Charlotte suffered from Dravet syndrome, a rare seizure disorder that cannot be controlled by existing medications. By the age of three, she was having three hundred grand mal seizures a week, and her family was low on options. Her heart had stopped multiple times and she lost the ability to eat, walk, and talk. Despite having voted against the legalization of marijuana, Charlotte's parents, desperate and willing to try just about anything, were able to get two physicians to sign off on a medical marijuana card for their daughter.

They heard through the grapevine that a low-THC, high-CBD strain of cannabis had helped another child suffering from the same disorder. So they got the card, purchased as much high-CBD medical cannabis as they could afford, and Charlotte became the youngest person ever in the medical marijuana program.

They had the high-CBD cannabis extracted and diluted in oil, and the first day they used it, Charlotte had no seizures. There were no seizures on the second, third, fifth, or seventh day either. Her parents were stunned, and also quickly running out of the high-CBD cannabis they had purchased. They learned that the Stanley brothers—who are well-known marijuana growers in Colorado—had developed a strain of marijuana that was high in CBD and low in THC but were having trouble selling it. The brothers heard Charlotte's story and agreed to help; they started a nonprofit called the Realm of Caring Foundation and started giving that high-CBD medical cannabis to patients suffering from a variety of different ailments.

Now, years later, Charlotte can walk, talk, and ride a bike, and is doing better than anyone expected. She has only a few seizures a month and still takes the Stanley brothers' strain of CBD oil (which is now named Charlotte's Web) in her food every single day. As you might expect, an explosion of public and political pressure to legalize the use of CBD oil, especially for patients like Charlotte, quickly followed. Many states started allowing for the "compassionate use" of CBD, which means that seriously ill patients can use CBD when no other treatment options are available.

CBD ENTERS THE WELLNESS SCENE

After Charlotte's story hit the airwaves, the potential health benefits of CBD were front of mind, and high-CBD strains of cannabis went from being practically unsellable to potentially lifesaving and in high demand. Wellness experts started wondering how they could use the compound not just to treat sick people but to keep healthy people healthy, relieve minor aches and pains we all experience daily, and potentially treat a group of disorders like IBS and anxiety that, like seizures, are characterized by "hyper-irritability" of bodily systems.

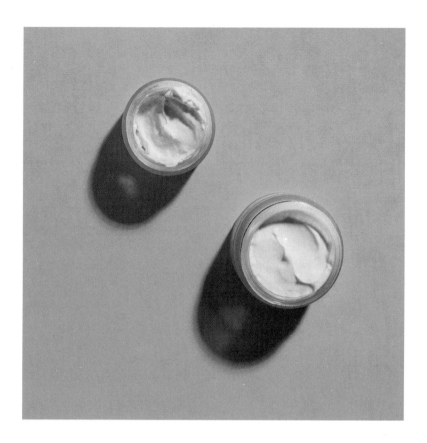

People love to criticize the wellness industry, and I have to say that the wellness industry doesn't make it all that hard. Society can admittedly get a little too caught up in the next big superfood or workout or smoothie-bowl recipe or cleanse or flower essence (I think you get the idea). But if we zoom out, wellness is pretty simple. It's about considering lifestyle changes before drugs, using food and exercise as preventive medicine (something that has been proven to work over and over and over again, by the way), and caring for the body as a whole instead of looking at it as a bunch of separate parts that each need their own specialist. The pillars of wellness are strong, and despite the fact that we can take things a little too far at times, there is no doubt in my mind that those smoothie bowls and trendy workouts are adding years to people's lives.

So now, just the way we've seen turmeric and coconut oil blow up every juice bar and café, we're now seeing CBD tonics, chocolates, and tinctures for sale at the same establishments. A popular Brooklyn café called The End, home of the famous Unicorn Latte (which if you haven't seen you should look up), started selling a CBD oil hot chocolate. People have realized that CBD has hundreds of potential skin-care applications and are wasting no time infusing it into soaps, face oils, and lotions to reap the benefits of its strong anti-inflammatory and antioxidant properties.

It's likely that your next question is: How are these people getting CBD oil when it's derived from cannabis? Well, the Stanley brothers and a bunch of other companies are selling CBD oil derived from *hemp*. Here's what that means and why they are able to do it without getting arrested.

THE LEGAL STATUS OF CBD

If you thought the science of CBD was complicated, just wait. The legal status of CBD is a real doozy, so I'll go over the basics and try not to get too lost in legal jargon—and keep in mind that the policies that govern CBD could change in an instant!

When it comes to the legality of marijuana, CBD, and hemp, we have to start with the Controlled Substances Act, which regulates and classifies substances that are intoxicating or have the potential to be abused. All substances are classified under one of five schedules, determined by balancing their potential benefits with their respective dangers. Then, the schedule to which they are assigned influences the rules and regulations that they are subject to.

Cannabis and the Controlled Substances Act

Under the Controlled Substances Act, the plant *Cannabis sativa*—which includes both hemp and marijuana, if you recall—is classified as a Schedule 1 substance. This means that it currently has no accepted medical use in the United States, a high potential for abuse, and a lack of accepted safety even under medical supervision. Accompanying cannabis on the list of Schedule 1 substances are drugs like heroin, LSD, ecstasy, methaqualone, and peyote. (Yes, really.)

Schedule 2 substances are different because they currently have "an accepted medical use" in the United States, though they are also described as having a high potential for abuse. Schedule 2 drugs include cocaine, methadone, oxycodone, fentanyl, Adderall, and Ritalin. Further down in the classification system are drugs in Schedule 3 (having a moderate to low potential for physical and psychological dependence) like ketamine, anabolic steroids, and testosterone; and Schedule 4 substances (having a low potential for abuse and low risk of dependence) like Xanax and Valium. The lowest ranked are Schedule 5 substances, which include drugs like cough syrups with codeine in them.

LEARNING WHAT HEMP REALLY IS

Now, obviously, many of us will take issue with the way these drugs have been classified, especially when it comes to cannabis. Any sane person would wonder how marijuana can be Schedule 1 while fentanyl, ketamine, and cocaine fall in Schedules 2 and 3. Many people will deny that there was any discrimination against cannabis when these drugs were classified—it's just that medications like morphine were already on the market in the 1970s when the Controlled Substances Act was enacted. In other words, because there was an FDA-approved opium-based drug (morphine), cocaine had no choice but to be labeled as Schedule 2, while cannabis defaulted to Schedule 1 because no cannabis-based drugs had been made yet. This may have been understandable at the time, but it begs the question: Why hasn't anything changed since? Sadly, it has proven really difficult to change a drug's classification, and many attempts to reschedule cannabis have failed during the legislative process or have been shot down in court.

Right now you might be thinking, *Hold on a second, I thought most CBD was derived from hemp, and hemp is legal, right?* You are right—hemp is legal in all fifty states and a legal US import, but that all depends on the actual definition of hemp itself. Legally, hemp plants are not defined by federal law. Instead, parts of the cannabis plant are simply exempted from the Schedule 1 substance classification. These parts include the stalks, fiber, and sterilized seeds, which have been used to make clothes and hempseed oil (not to be confused with hemp oil) for many years.

So what does this mean? It means that the whole hemp plant is defined as marijuana under law. Therefore, to make a truly hemp-derived CBD product, you can extract CBD only from the stalks of the plant. The problem with this is that that these parts of the plant aren't abundant in cannabinoids, which is why they were exempted from the Schedule 1 substance classification in the first place. Cannabinoids are largely located in the flowering portions of the plant, expressed in golf ball–like structures called *trichomes*. This is problematic for hemp-based CBD manufacturers: Do they extract from only the stalks and seeds, which typically creates a product that has questionable potency and quality, or do they extract from the whole plant (including the flowering portion) even though technically it then qualifies as a Schedule 1 substance?

Thus far, I've been talking about federal laws, but there are also state laws governing CBD. Sadly, it doesn't get any less complicated at this point. You might be surprised to learn that the first state to pass a CBD law and become a "CBD state" was Alabama, which passed legislation in 2014 legalizing CBD products for people with rare seizure disorders. Other states quickly followed suit and passed their own version of this law, which allows for cannabis extracts to be used for people with specific medical conditions as long as the extracts are low enough in THC. Sadly, there isn't any real standardization of these laws, and each state seemed to just create its own version, so the exact regulations are all over the place.

In states that have medical marijuana laws, CBD is lawful, but you have to get a recommendation from a health care professional, and most states limit access to CBD to patients with certain qualifying conditions like glaucoma or seizure disorders. In states where cannabis is legal for recreational use, you can access CBD easily, and it's legal to have no matter what kind of cannabis plant it's made from.

Then the Agricultural Act of 2014 (also known as the Farm Bill) was passed. This bill authorized certain institutions to grow industrialized hemp for research, as long as the state law permitted it. In this bill, industrial hemp is defined as *Cannabis sativa* having a THC concentration that is less than 0.3 percent. You'll see the magic number 0.3 percent all over the place as what differentiates hemp from marijuana, and as the legal basis for being able to sell CBD oil nationwide. But as I just described, when it comes to the definition of hemp, this number is somewhat trivial since hemp is also defined as specific parts of the cannabis plant. In addition, this law isn't all that specific about what *research* really means, so some states and companies are interpreting it in a way that allows them to authorize certain independent growers to grow "hemp" and then sell the products commercially as long as they are less than 0.3 percent THC.

I could talk about this all day, but the take-home message here is that many CBD oil companies are operating in a legal gray area, and this is made possible by the lack of specificity in the laws that govern and define hemp. It doesn't seem like anyone—from the Food and Drug Administration (FDA) to the Drug Enforcement Administration to the CBD oil manufacturers to the patients—knows what the best way to define CBD in terms of safety, regulation, legality, and continued access actually is.

All this being said, CBD companies operating within currently accepted parameters are selling CBD products nationwide without significant interference. That could change in the future, but so far there has been no significant enforcement against consumers or vendors for selling CBD or hemp oil as long as it is nonintoxicating and made from a plant with less than 0.3 percent THC.

CBD AND SUPPLEMENT REGULATIONS (OR LACK THEREOF)

Phew, are you happy that part's over? I am. It's really confusing, and one can easily get lost in the nitty-gritty details and technicalities. But if we take a step back, the reality is that whether or not buying and selling and taking hemp-based CBD oil is entirely legal, people are buying it and selling it and taking it. That begs the very important question: How are these products being regulated?

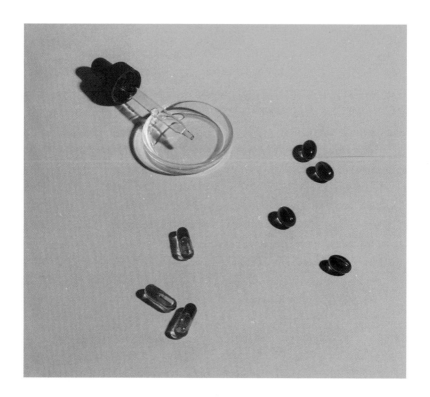

Here, CBD falls in a gray area once again. This is because currently, CBD is regulated a lot like a supplement, and when it comes to regulating supplements, it's largely up to the supplement company itself to set its own quality standards and to follow them. At the end of the day, the manufacturers of dietary supplements are in charge of making sure their products are safe, effective, and labeled properly. They are not reviewed by the government before they go to market but the FDA is responsible for investigating adverse reports and can take action if they are able to prove that supplement company has been making false or misleading claims.

The FDA also scours the websites, promotional material, and labels of supplements to make sure there aren't any unlawful statements or medical claims, like that an herb can cure or heal a specific disease, for example. Therefore, there is some *semblance* of regulation, but when you buy a supplement or a CBD oil, you are definitely putting a *lot* of faith in the company that makes it, sources it, and labels it.

In 2015, the FDA issued warning letters to six CBD companies saying that they were making medical claims on their respective websites, labels, or social media accounts. They did the same thing to eight more companies in 2016 and to four more in 2017. During this evaluation, the FDA also lab tested many of these products and found that some of them didn't contain the amounts of CBD stated on the label, and in some cases, they didn't contain any CBD at all.

Knowing this, if you read only one chapter in this book, make it chapter 8, on finding a good CBD product. It will give you some guidelines for what questions to ask before you buy, including how to find a brand that goes above and beyond to make sure they're selling—and you're buying—a high-quality product.

5

The Health Benefits of CBD

I'm a writer and admittedly obsessed with most things health and wellness, but first and foremost I'm a scientist. That means that when I see something touted as a miracle remedy or superfood, my first thought is, *That's unlikely*, and my first response is, "Show me the research." When it comes to supplements and natural remedies, it's so important to take a long, hard look at the evidence and evaluate it with a critical eye. That being said, you don't want to be overly critical or closed-minded, because you'll miss out on a lot. This balance between skepticism and receptivity is critical when evaluating the benefits of CBD, but before I show you the research, I want to talk a little bit about research in general. Bear with me!

WHAT "SCIENTIFIC EVIDENCE" REALLY MEANS

To put it simply: There are a *lot* of different types of research. And saying that something is supported by science can mean any number of different things. First, there are in vitro studies, which are mostly conducted in test tubes and Petri dishes and are mainly used to observe the activity of CBD on a microscopic level or in a controlled environment instead of in a living organism. Then there are animal studies, which can give researchers helpful hints as to how a substance will react in humans. These aren't foolproof, as certain treatments can work very differently in humans than they do in animals. There are review papers, which analyze a bunch of studies on the same topic to figure out what the overall consensus is; and there are observational studies, where scientists observe the health and behavior of groups of people for a specific amount of time. There's also anecdotal evidence, and this includes case studies or stories like Charlotte's. Science sometimes likes to dismiss pieces of anecdotal evidence as flukes, coincidences, or isolated incidences—but other times scientists listen up and allow these stories to guide the direction of their research. I'm happy to report that since Charlotte's story broke, there have been multiple studies on the effects of CBD on seizure disorders.

And finally, there are clinical trials, which evaluate the effectiveness of a treatment in humans in a very specific way. There are a lot of different types of clinical trials, but the gold standard research model is the double-blind placebo-controlled randomized controlled trial (try saying that ten times fast). These studies go something like this: Scientists isolate a specific treatment (in this case, CBD oil) and test it on populations of people, who have been randomly assigned to different groups, for a very specific amount of time. Some groups would get the actual CBD treatment, and others would get a fake treatment, but none of the participants in the study or the practitioners evaluating them for changes in their condition would know if they got the real treatment or the fake one. This is all meant to decrease bias from the researchers and the likelihood that the placebo effect will skew the patients' results. These studies are well designed to eliminate all factors that could affect the participant outcomes except for the factor that researchers actually want to know more about.

This is both brilliant and frustrating. Think about it for a second: How do you study acupuncture under this research model? Or an herbal remedy that requires the patient to see, smell, and taste the herb?

The Western research model works amazingly well in some cases, but it doesn't leave much room for adaptation, especially to more alternative ways of approaching medicine, which are oftentimes hands-on and more personalized. This is further complicated in cases like CBD, with its absurdly wide range of therapeutic properties. What benefit do you study first and on whom?

It comes as a surprise to many, but randomized controlled trials *have* been performed on CBD. And this is great, but it's far from proof that CBD has all the benefits wellness experts suspect it does. This is because the way the scientific community looks at it, unless you and I fit the profile of the participants in the study, the results from that study don't say much about how CBD oil will work for us. You can't assume that because CBD showed antianxiety effects in rats, it'll show the same in humans. You can't assume that if CBD works for a certain type of seizure disorder in children, it'll work for all people with seizures. Basically, you can't assume anything, ever.

If you hadn't noticed yet, I'm really into science. But I'm also a writer, and therefore I know that, beyond a shadow of a doubt, there is nothing more powerful than a story. When I started talking to people about their experiences with CBD oil, the first-person stories—from people whose lives have been changed by CBD—were by far the most compelling. And that's why I decided to include three in this book. These cases aren't medical proof of CBD's powers, nor do they guarantee that you will have the same success. But they do tell the stories of people who went from struggling with severe pain, taking multiple medications, or going days without sleep to living a better life, thanks at least in part to CBD. These stories are fair, and they range from "CBD saved my life" to "It was one piece of the larger puzzle that was reclaiming my health." These people want you to know that they are happy they turned to CBD.

So what does the existing science say about CBD? Now that you have all that highly important background information, I will finally tell you. Here's a big list of the different benefits of CBD. All of them are supported by *some* type of research or strong anecdotal evidence provided by multiple patients, clinicians, and health care providers. In other words, there is some reason to believe that CBD might help with the following.

CBD, Inflammation, and Autoimmune Disease

From inflammation-fighting workouts and self-care practices to the anti-inflammatory food pyramid, the health and wellness industries are obsessed with inflammation. I'm here to tell you that it's for good reason! Inflammation plays a massive role in health and disease. That's why, by far, the most exciting thing about CBD is its potential to help with chronic inflammation and autoimmune disease. If you're not sure what this means, don't worry. You're about to learn some of the basics about inflammation and autoimmune diseases, from a holistic health perspective, how they're related, and why they're such a big problem today.

Understanding Inflammation and Autoimmunity

Let's start with the very important fact that inflammation is a completely normal (and healthy!) response in the body designed to protect us from harm. For example, if you hit your knee, it might become red and swollen. This is the result of your immune system triggering an inflammatory response that sends special cells to protect the area. Without inflammation, simple infections or injuries could be much more dangerous—and even deadly. So we can all thank our bodies for creating acute inflammation when it's really needed.

So what's the problem with inflammation then? The short answer is that inflammation becomes a problem when it is chronic. Chronic underlying inflammation plays a role in an absurd number of conditions, many of which you will recognize as the biggest threats facing people's health today (think heart disease, cancer, dementia, depression, and type 2 diabetes). Chronic inflammation is also connected to widespread conditions like asthma, which is characterized by inflammation of the airways, and arthritis, which is inflammation of the joints that causes pain and stiffness. Scientists even have reason to believe that one of the major factors in depression is inflammation in the brain. Dr. Andrew Luster of the Center for Immunology and Inflammatory Diseases at Harvard-affiliated Massachusetts General Hospital described inflammation as "a smoldering process that injures your tissues, joints, and blood vessels, and you often do not notice it until significant damage is done." Sounds fun, right?

The consequences of inflammation vary, but leading integrative medicine doctors believe that if inflammation is allowed to fester for too long it can turn into an autoimmune disease. Autoimmune diseases are a group of conditions characterized by a paradigm shift in the immune system when it starts to register the body's own tissue as a threat. There are over a hundred different autoimmune diseases out there, but all of them involve the immune system attacking a different part of the body as if it were a pathogen or dangerous invader. Some examples of classic autoimmune disorders are rheumatoid arthritis, multiple sclerosis, inflammatory bowel diseases like Crohn's and ulcerative colitis, thyroid conditions like Hashimoto's or Graves' disease, and skin conditions like psoriasis and eczema.

What are the consequences of these illnesses? Well, that depends on whom you ask. When you're diagnosed with an autoimmune disease by conventional medicine doctors, they'll most likely tell you that you'll have the disease for life and your treatment will be all about *managing* your symptoms, normally using drugs like immunomodulatory medications and steroids. Integrative and functional medicine doctors, on the other hand, pride themselves on being able to manage and even reverse (in some cases) these diseases with diet, lifestyle changes, and herbs and supplements that help your body decrease inflammation and bring balance back to your immune system. Typically, they won't consider your autoimmune symptoms a life sentence, and CBD is likely on their list of natural remedies to employ to help you get your life back.

How to Know If You're at Risk for Chronic Inflammation

So how do you know if this "smoldering process" is occurring inside your body? If you visit an integrative or functional medicine doctor, he or she might run some lab tests, but even more likely, the doctor will ask you a bunch of questions about how you're feeling, since your body sends some very helpful hints when it's chronically inflamed. According to leading integrative and functional medicine experts, some tell-tale signs that chronic inflammation is a problem for you include:

- Chronic fatigue
- Accumulation of fat around the abdomen and trouble maintaining your weight
- Digestive issues like gas, diarrhea, bloating, or constipation
- Skin issues like rashes or itchiness
- Worsening seasonal allergies
- Chronic brain fog or frequent headaches
- Anxiety or depression
- Chronic pain or achiness
- Trouble sleeping or staying asleep

Do any of these apply to you? If the answer is yes (and it will be for most of us), we're presented with a choice: We can think of these symptoms as everyday health woes and cover them up with over-the-counter medicines, or we can consider them small warning signs from the body that something about our diet and lifestyle needs adjusting.

So how do we fight inflammation? You start by getting advice by a health care provider who is well versed in inflammation. But we'll cover the basics here, and that starts with avoiding the stuff that causes inflammation and filling your days with the stuff that lessens it.

Things That Cause Inflammation

- Smoking
- Alcohol (in excess)
- Sugar and artificial sweeteners
- Refined grains (like those in most white bread, pasta, cakes, and cookies)
- Fried and processed foods
- Toxic chemicals in our air, food, water, environment, cosmetics, and household and cleaning products (think BPA and parabens)
- Red meat, especially processed meats like lunch meat and sausages

- Unhealthy fats like soybean and canola oil as well as all hydrogenated oils
- Dairy products like milk, cheese, and ice cream
- An imbalanced gut microbiome (this means too many bad bacteria in the gastrointestinal tract and not enough good ones)
- Too much exercise
- Too little exercise
- Chronic stress
- Lack of sleep

Things That Fight Inflammation
- Healthy fats like olive oil, fatty fish like salmon, nuts, and seeds
- Colorful fruits and vegetables (especially berries and leafy green vegetables) with plenty of healthy fiber
- Superfoods like turmeric and green tea
- Meditation, yoga, and other mindfulness-based stress-reduction techniques
- At least seven hours of sleep a night; some people need nine

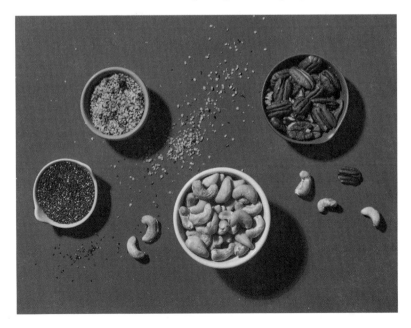

- The right amount of exercise for your body
- Spending time in nature
- Fermented foods like sauerkraut and probiotics, which contain beneficial bacteria for the gut

You'll notice that the recipes in this book are formulated with a ton of inflammation-fighting and antioxidant-rich foods and ingredients. This is done on purpose, because fighting inflammation and promoting longevity isn't just about living your life and adding CBD oil to the mix— it's about living an anti-inflammatory lifestyle and using CBD oil to complement your other healthy endeavors. The reality is this: You can't CBD oil your way out of a crappy diet and lifestyle routine. That's the part you have to figure out first, which is why this book is a full lifestyle manual, not just a book about how to take CBD.

The Anti-Inflammatory Properties of CBD

Now that you're an expert on inflammation, I'm going to tell you how CBD could be helpful in your quest to lower chronic inflammation. It starts with the fact that the endocannabinoid system (ECS) is intricately involved in the body's inflammatory response. As I mentioned before, endocannabinoids temper excess activity in the body, and this can really help bring the inflammatory response back to balance by inhibiting cell proliferation (a process where cells divide and multiply rapidly) and suppressing cytokine production and eicosanoid signaling (which are both complex processes that contribute to inflammation in the body). Cannabinoids also work to induce regulatory T cells, which help the immune system distinguish between the body's own tissue and foreign invaders, which, as we now know, is the hallmark of preventing autoimmune disease.

On top of all this, we know that endocannabinoid signaling is altered when there's persistent inflammation in the body, which further confirms that the ECS interacts directly with the inflammatory process. Researchers are playing with the idea that cannabinoids could help treat a wide range of inflammatory disorders, and some even suspect cannabinoids will become a whole new family of anti-inflammatory drugs. This is great news for people with autoimmune and inflammatory illnesses, as the existing treatment options can leave them choosing between the symptoms of their disease and the side effects of their medication. Those people deserve more options.

CBD and Mental Health

CBD is quickly gaining fame and recognition for its antianxiety properties, but anxiety isn't the only mental health condition for which CBD shows promise. Currently, CBD is being explored as a possible treatment for anxiety, depression, post-traumatic stress disorder, bipolar disorder, and even schizophrenia. Why the strong connection to mental health? Well, the ECS is intricately involved in the activities in our brains that govern mood, and many researchers suspect that when our endocannabinoid tone is low, we're more likely to experience mental health instability and mood-related disorders.

How CBD Works in the Brain

So how does CBD work in the brain, exactly? Let's start off by saying that the brain works in strange and mysterious ways. The cells in the brain—called *neurons*—form complex networks, and one of the ways they communicate with each other is by releasing chemical messengers called *neurotransmitters*, which are largely in charge of our moods and emotional responses. These neurotransmitters swim around the brain and match up with various receptors where they can attach and create a desired effect (like making us feel happy or bonded to our partners). This is important because cannabinoids can also interact with these receptors and create similar responses or change the response that's occurring.

One of the most interesting ways CBD influences our mental health is through its ability to bind directly to the 5-HT_{1A} serotonin receptor, which is known to govern anxiety and depression. People with these conditions often have low levels of serotonin, and serotonin itself regulates things like appetite, nausea, sleep, mood, anxiety, and pain perception. This receptor is also the target for selective serotonin reuptake inhibitors, which are one of the major classes of antidepressant medications.

Another important neurotransmitter is called GABA, and it works to inhibit brain cell activity, making it useful in the treatment of anxiety. If you suffer from anxiety, you can probably relate to the feeling of just wanting to turn your brain off. Enhancing the effect of GABA in the brain is the main action of benzodiazepines, which are the most common antianxiety medications and include drugs like Xanax and Klonopin. CBD has been shown to act directly on $GABA_A$ receptors in a way that changes their shape and increases GABA's effects.

Last but not least, chronic stress and anxiety cause an enzyme in the body called *fatty acid amide hydrolase* (FAAH) to spin out of control. When this happens, it can hurt endocannabinoid tone. Luckily, studies have shown that CBD can inhibit the FAAH enzyme, protecting our bodies from the damaging effects of chronic stress, which can cause, exacerbate, or at least play a role in most mental health conditions.

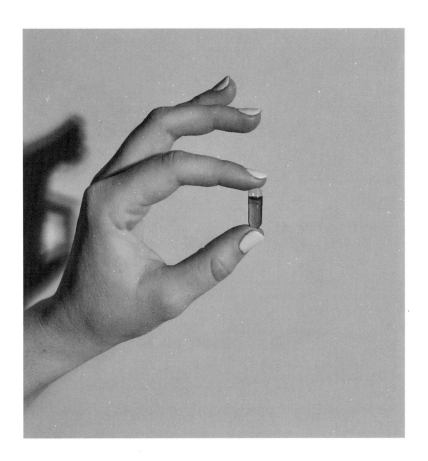

CBD and Anxiety, Depression, and PTSD

I was happy to discover that there's pretty good scientific evidence to back up the idea that CBD can help with anxiety. In animal studies, CBD has been shown to fight measures of stress and anxiety. It's also been shown to abate public-speaking-induced anxiety and symptoms of generalized anxiety disorder in human trials. Still, there has yet to be a definitive clinical trial on CBD's true potential as an antianxiety remedy. Luckily, it looks like they are on the way: the first big clinical study on the effects of CBD on adults with anxiety is due to begin in 2018 at a hospital in Massachusetts.

When it comes to CBD and depression, many experts and users of

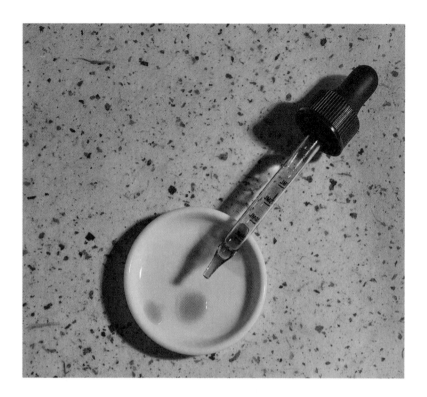

CBD oil say it boosts mood almost immediately. Right now, the scientific evidence connecting CBD and depression consists mostly of the studies I mentioned earlier, which connect the activity and tone of the endocannabinoid system to mood issues. Studies have also shown that people with depression often have lower levels of AEA and 2-AG than people without it. This is a start, but there's still a lot we need to learn. In the coming years, researchers in Brazil will look at CBD as an adjunctive treatment for bipolar depression; researchers suspect they will observe significant improvement in depression, anxiety, and also inflammation (which, as I mentioned, is proving to be a factor in depression).

One of the other exciting avenues of CBD research has to do with post-traumatic stress disorder, more often referred to as PTSD. This is a condition that develops after a person experiences or witnesses a traumatic event and is characterized by reliving the event, engaging in avoidance behaviors, and experiencing panic attacks, depression, and suicidal thoughts. It's particularly common in the veteran community, and many people struggle with it for years, bouncing from one psychiatric medication to another, never finding significant relief.

There have been quite a few anecdotal stories of veterans who were able to trade an entire medicine cabinet full of prescription drugs—and all the side effects that come with them—for medical marijuana, and it would make sense that CBD (with its soothing and antipsychotic properties) would be the cannabinoid of choice for treating PTSD. One study analyzed people who were near the World Trade Center on 9/11 and found that those who developed PTSD from the event had lower levels of the endogenous cannabinoid AEA; this is part of a larger trend that shows that people who develop PTSD generally have a low endocannabinoid tone. Martin Lee, in an article about the connection between PTSD and the ECS, wrote, "PTSD is one of many enigmatic conditions that may arise because of a dysfunctional endocannabinoid system."

CBD and Psychiatric Medications

CBD works on similar parts of the brain as common psychiatric medications like selective serotonin reuptake inhibitors or benzodiazepines, so why not just use the pharmaceutical medications that you can get at the pharmacy? That's a valid question. First, let's look at benzodiazepines, the most common form of antianxiety medications.

Benzos, as they're often called, are highly addictive and very dangerous when abused, especially when mixed with alcohol (think roofies). For frequent users, there is a list of side effects so long it's *almost* comical until you read it and realize that "coma" and "confusion about identity, place, and time" are all on the list. When you go off of these commonly prescribed drugs (Xanax being the third most commonly prescribed psychiatric medication in the United States), there is a long list of withdrawal symptoms, including—but not limited to—convulsions, hallucinations, headaches, stomach or muscle cramps, tremors, and trouble sleeping.

Now, let's be clear, I don't want to vilify these drugs, and I'd never say they're inherently bad or unnecessary; in fact, I've used them, and they've been a lifesaver. That being said, I can't ignore their risks—especially when it comes to chronic use and abuse—and I have to be fair when I compare their safety profile to that of CBD, which has no known serious negative side effects or withdrawal symptoms documented so far. The biggest problem is that researchers don't know enough about how well CBD works to directly compare it to benzos or consider it a substitute.

When it comes to depression, the two most common drugs are Zoloft and Celexa (these are also the two most commonly prescribed psychiatric drugs in general). Unfortunately, there are a lot of questions about how well these go-to prescription medications actually work, especially for milder forms of depression. Research has shown that the more severe one's depression is, the more likely depression medications are to help. And even then, an article published in 2017 by the Institute for Quality and Efficiency in Healthcare showed that only about twenty out of a hundred people with moderate to severe depression will experience improved symptoms with medication.

Meanwhile, more than half of all people taking antidepressants experience side effects. These can be milder, like dry mouth, headaches, and loss of sex drive, or they can be more serious, like liver damage or nausea or dizziness so severe it leads to falls. Again, I would never say that these medications are inherently bad. They can be lifesaving for many, many, many people. What I'm saying—and I don't think any doctor would disagree—is that there's a lot of room for improvement. So regardless of whether or not CBD becomes more important when it comes to depression, we should be tirelessly searching for treatment options that are more effective than the ones we have.

CBD and Brain Health

When it comes to brain health, CBD's antioxidant, neuroprotective, and anti-inflammatory properties are paramount. Multiple scientific studies, including one published in the journal *Free Radical Biology and Medicine*, have shown that CBD does indeed work to prevent free radical damage, reduce inflammation, and protect the brain cells. A review paper published in the *British Journal of Pharmacology* titled "The Role of Cannabinoids in Pharmacology" also describes CBD's ability to stimulate neurogenesis, which is a word used to describe the growth of new brain cells.

So what does this mean for us? It means that CBD may be a good addition to certain wellness regimes focused on supporting brain health, and that it could potentially be used to help heal the brain after concussions or traumatic brain injuries. These types of injuries are the result of trauma to the head, and short-term symptoms include pain and dizziness. Many patients, however, experience long-term chronic problems like an inability to focus, memory issues, or anxiety and depression. The University of Miami received a large grant to study the effects of cannabinoids on traumatic brain injuries and concussions, which researchers think will help decrease inflammation and the overactive immune response in the brain that occurs after injury. Healing from these kinds of injuries is a slow, arduous process, but there's reason to think that CBD could support people as they go through it.

When we're talking about brain health, it's impossible not to mention neurodegenerative diseases like Alzheimer's and Parkinson's disease, which are becoming more prevalent every day. Parkinson's, in particular, is characterized by a deficiency in dopamine (another important neurotransmitter in the brain), and interestingly, research has shown that CBD is able to boost dopamine levels. A small study has already shown that CBD can improve quality of life for people with Parkinson's. When it comes to Alzheimer's, studies—including one published in the *International Journal of Molecular Sciences* titled "Cannabidiol Modulates the Expression of Alzheimer's Disease-Related Genes in Mesenchymal Stem Cells"—have shown that CBD can help prevent the formation of plaques that mark the development of the disease. A study published in the journal *Nature Medicine* showed that cannabinoid therapy was also able to improve memory and cognition in mice.

We also know that neurodegenerative conditions like Alzheimer's and Parkinson's have a strong lifestyle component, meaning that the food we eat, our level of activity, and how we live our lives matters—a lot. In fact, in some circles Alzheimer's is referred to as Type 3 diabetes. One factor in particular, gut health, seems to play a particularly strong role. Research shows that the diversity and strength of the bacteria in the gut can be linked to the development of neurodegenerative diseases like Alzheimer's, as well as to depression, which is one more reason to read the section on gut health. Luckily, that section is coming up right about now.

CBD and Gut Health

Hippocrates, the father of modern medicine, said that "all disease begins in the gut," and he could not have been more right. If you're into wellness, you know that pretty much everything we do is aimed at improving gut health. Why, you ask? Besides the fact that bloating, diarrhea, constipation, and stomach pain are all day ruiners, we're finding more and more that the communities of bacteria living in our digestive tract rule a lot of different aspects of our health—everything from our energy levels to our mood to the strength of our immune system to our ability to lose weight and absorb nutrients from our food. All of that sounds pretty important, doesn't it?

There are a few different gut health issues that get a lot of attention, and one of them is something referred to as leaky gut. Leaky gut occurs when the tight junctions of the small intestines become damaged, mostly due to a poor diet, certain medications, and stress. As a result, these junctions—which are supposed to act like gates between the gastrointestinal tract and bloodstream—become less discerning about what is absorbed. This increased permeability allows food particles and other unmentionables to sneak through the intestinal wall and into the bloodstream, where they wreak havoc, in the form of chronic inflammation, on our bodies. Increased intestinal permeability has been linked to a bunch of different illnesses and disorders including allergies, metabolic disease, and irritable bowel syndrome (IBS). So what does this have to do with CBD? Scientists think that cannabidiol might be able to act directly on these tight junctions to help them function more efficiently. This means increased absorption of nutrients you want in your body— and fewer particles slipping through that aren't supposed to be there.

Another common digestive health issue is IBS, which comes with a host of undesirable symptoms. IBS is extremely common; I'd be surprised if you couldn't name at least one person who has it. CBD's antispasmodic properties and anti-inflammatory properties make it an attractive option for treating irritable bowel syndrome, but we're also finding that IBS flare-ups are linked to stress, which means that CBD might help with IBS in more ways than one. Quite a few case reports and preclinical studies have strongly suggested that CBD could provide those suffering from IBS some relief, so now we're just waiting on those pesky clinical studies. Luckily, there's a clinical trial in the works in the Netherlands that will test the effects of CBD-containing chewing gum on irritable bowel syndrome.

CBD and Pain

Pain isn't something we think about until we're experiencing it, and then we can't get it off our minds. But if you take a second to look around, you'll see that pain is everywhere. People are suffering from acute pain conditions like back pain or postsurgery pain and lifelong diseases that cause chronic pain like multiple sclerosis and fibromyalgia. A lot of people are using CBD oil to treat all kinds of pain—and they swear by it. This is great news, since the current treatment options (ahem, opioids) can have dangerous side effects and a very high risk for addiction.

CBD, THC, and Pain

So how does CBD work to fight pain? The analgesic properties of cannabis have long been attributed to THC, which we know can reduce pain all on its own; a drug called Sativex (with a 1:1 CBD-to-THC ratio) has even been approved in Europe and Canada to treat certain types of pain—like cancer-related pain—that are often unresponsive to opioids. Therefore, we know that THC can fight pain on its own and that a CBD-THC combo is also effective, but can CBD fight pain on its own? And if so, how does it work?

CBD does seem to be able to reduce pain all on its own—one study even showed that a topical cannabidiol preparation could improve arthritic pain in animals—but we're not entirely sure how effective it is without the entourage effect provided by higher levels of THC than you can get in any hemp-based CBD oils. Scientists hypothesize that CBD's pain-fighting properties have a lot to do with its anti-inflammatory activity and how it interacts with certain receptors in the brain.

How CBD Fights Pain in the Body

To get specific, CBD interacts with a family of receptors called *vanilloid receptors* that mediate pain perception, inflammation levels, and even body temperature. CBD has been shown to activate a specific receptor called *vanilloid type 1 receptor* (TRPV1), which is known to play a role in inflammatory pain. Capsaicin—the strong, spicy compound in hot chile peppers—has long been used as an alternative treatment for pain, and it also activates the TRPV1 receptor. (Cue the Chile Cheese Popcorn recipe on page 139, which combines the pain-fighting properties of both CBD and capsaicin.)

The use of cannabinoids to treat chronic pain is one of the most exciting areas of research and has the potential to change the way we treat pain in America. And if you know anything about the current state of the opioid epidemic, you know that a lot needs to change. Available pain medications and pain-modulating procedures are extremely limited by their low efficacy and high toxicity, safety concerns, inaccessibility, and high costs.

Research shows that CBD and opioids work very differently in the body, so they could potentially be used in combination to tag team chronic pain. However, a study on over three thousand patients conducted by UC Berkeley and HelloMD—a digital health care platform for the cannabis industry—showed that 81 percent of patients "agree" or "strongly agree" that cannabis by itself was more effective than taking cannabis and opioids together. So the jury is out for now. There is currently a study being performed by the University of Utah that will test cannabinoid-based therapies (including one high-CBD and low-THC therapy) on patients who suffer from chronic pain. The researchers plan to get a better idea of any risks and side effects of the treatments and also to identify any changes that occur in the brain throughout the study period.

CBD and Insomnia

CBD is often touted as an amazing treatment for insomnia, but as I mentioned before, there's also evidence that CBD has a wakening and energizing effect. In fact, some people refer to it as a stimulant or "waking agent," and it might interact with the same receptors in the brain as caffeine. That being said, some studies suggest it can help improve sleep duration and quality. Yes, I know it's contradictory and not as cut-and-dried as what people struggling to sleep want to hear.

So does CBD help with sleep or not? I asked a lot of CBD experts about this one, and the conclusion I've reached is that CBD's ability to help with sleep disorders depends on both the dosage and *why* a person can't sleep. If insomnia is anxiety induced, which it frequently is, CBD is more likely to help calm the mind before bed and get the person to sleep. If a person has disrupted sleep for another reason, it's definitely worth experimenting with CBD, but that person might ultimately find that CBD isn't the best choice.

If you're taking CBD for insomnia, it's really important to experiment with different doses, and even CBD-to-THC ratios if you live in a state with recreational or medical marijuana. And while it's always a good idea to consult an expert before trying CBD, this is a situation where it's especially important to work with a doctor or health care professional well versed in the science of cannabidiol and sleep.

CBD and Serious Medical Conditions

Seizures

As we know from Charlotte's story, one of the most groundbreaking implications for CBD has to do with epileptic disorders, especially diseases like Lennox-Gastaut syndrome and Dravet syndrome, which are unresponsive to medication. Seizure disorders, in general, are famously hard to treat, and learning this makes the fact that the anti-seizure properties of CBD have been known for decades but barely studied until recently particularly hard to swallow.

How effective is CBD for seizures, really? In 2016, a study showed that CBD-rich medical cannabis led to a reduction in seizure frequency in 89 percent of the participants. In 2012, GW Pharmaceuticals started researching the anti-seizure properties of CBD and began clinical trials on a new drug called Epidiolex. Epidiolex is a purified, 99 percent oil-based CBD extract from the cannabis plant (made from the flowering part of the plant, then put through an extraction process to remove the THC). It is already approved in Europe and received final approval by the FDA in 2018—the first drug in the United States extracted from cannabis.

Once it's out, many patients who have been using hemp-based CBD products will have to decide whether or not to switch to the more pharmaceutical route or stick with the whole-plant extracts they've been buying from dispensaries or online. Many of them have had such success with the hemp-based products that they're not planning on disrupting their treatment protocols.

A few other pharmaceutical companies are developing synthetic CBD for different kinds of epilepsy; one is a transdermal gel and the other is an oral solution. Hopefully, in the near future, we will understand exactly how CBD works to reduce seizures and have a better understanding of its long-term safety—especially in children whose brains are still developing.

Addiction

It might seem ironic to talk about CBD—which is technically a Schedule 1 substance—in the context of fighting addiction. But knowing more about the science of CBD, you probably aren't surprised by the idea that CBD is being considered by doctors and researchers as a potential complementary treatment for addiction symptoms. There are quite a few types of addiction that CBD might help with, but since I just talked about pain, I'll tackle opioid addiction first.

Let's start off with this fact: In states where medical marijuana is legal, there has been an almost 25 percent drop in opioid-related overdoses. That number feels significant, but when you consider the fact that over 65,000 people die every year from opioid-related overdoses, your jaw might hit the floor. And while experts hope to use CBD as a pain therapy in place of opioids, but it's so much more than that. Research has suggested that CBD could also help reduce the opioid dosage needed by chronic pain sufferers, lessen withdrawal symptoms from coming off opioids, and at the very least, become a treatment option to try before opioids are prescribed in the first place.

High on the list of devastating addictions is alcoholism. Yes, as strange as it is, we're about to talk about using an illegal substance to help people who are addicted to a legal one. Over 80,000 deaths a year can be attributed to alcohol in some way, and overdoses are extremely common. Cannabis, on the other hand, has a very low risk of overdose or death. To be more specific: *No deaths have ever been directly attributed to consuming too much cannabis.* Again and again, the science has shown that cannabis is not only safer than alcohol, it could actually be a way to prevent and treat alcohol abuse.

Interestingly, there's also reason to believe that the anti-inflammatory and antioxidant properties of CBD may protect the body from the detrimental effects of alcohol abuse. A recent study showed that alcoholics who were also frequent marijuana smokers were less likely to develop liver disease. Research also suggests that cannabis can help people detox from alcohol use by interacting with receptors and neurotransmitters in the brain that make withdrawal and sobriety more manageable. Most of this research has been done on combination CBD-THC remedies, so there's still a lot to learn about CBD alone and alcoholism.

But what about marijuana—isn't it addictive? Researchers are finding that marijuana, specifically the mind-altering effects from THC, can be "addictive" in some sense of the word, but not in a way that is seriously harmful to users or to the world around them compared to other drugs or substances. The side effects of marijuana withdrawal are unpleasant, but not necessarily severe—at least, not compared to other drugs. In the documentary miniseries *Weed* by Sanjay Gupta, an expert explains that withdrawing from THC is much more about withdrawing from the social habits you have built around it.

As far as researchers can tell, the "addictive" qualities of cannabis do not seem to have much to do with CBD, and so CBD oil is currently being tested as a way to wean people off THC if they are frequent marijuana users and they feel that it's negatively affecting their life. CBD has been described in multiple scientific studies as an "anti-addictive compound."

So when will we know more about the effects of CBD on addiction? A study is currently being conducted at the NYU School of Medicine that will test the effects of CBD on treating alcohol use disorder in individuals suffering from PTSD. Other studies are evaluating the effects of CBD on cocaine cravings and relapse from cocaine addiction. Clearly, there are a ton of reasons to believe that CBD can help reduce the use of prescription drugs, recreational drugs, alcohol, and in some cases even THC.

Cancer

There's no arguing that cancer is one of the biggest threats to our health. In fact, the CDC predicts that there will be 1.9 million new cancer diagnoses in 2020 in the United States alone. When researchers began studying the potential benefits of CBD for cancer, they were mostly focused on minimizing cancer-treatment-related symptoms like nausea from chemotherapy or pain from radiation. In fact, there's already a THC-inspired drug on the market for use during chemotherapy, and there's a lot of evidence that the endocannabinoid system regulates nausea and vomiting. Many, many people have found CBD helpful throughout their cancer-treatment process. (Just remember to always talk to your doctor before adding anything to your treatment protocol.)

Surprisingly, CBD might actually slow the growth of cancer itself. Various in vitro studies have shown that CBD helps encourage cancer cells to die, and animal studies have shown that CBD may slow the growth and spread of certain types of cancers. Right now, CBD and other cannabinoids are being tested on humans in various clinical trials, and the results are promising—showing increased cancer cell death, decreased tumor growth, and inhibition of metastasis (which is when cancer cells spread to other parts of the body). In addition, scientists at the California Pacific Medical Center Research Institute have discovered that CBD inhibits breast cancer metastasis and are now researching the role CBD might be able to play in slowing the progression of one of the most aggressive forms of brain cancer.

How is all this possible? I probably sound like a broken record by now, but scientists are postulating that this ability has everything to do with CBD's antioxidant and anti-inflammatory properties. Keep in mind, these studies use CBD as a complementary treatment to chemotherapy, radiation, surgery, and other *approved medical treatments* for cancer. We are a long way from even considering the idea that CBD could become a replacement for any of these lifesaving interventions.

CBD and Your Pet

If you thought the benefits of CBD were limited to humans, you'll be happy to know that the Internet is full of uplifting stories about pet owners turning to CBD oil to help their furry friends. Pets can suffer from many of the same health woes—from seizure disorders and arthritis to erratic behavior and separation anxiety—as humans. Most of this evidence is anecdotal at the minute, but more and more veterinarians are suggesting CBD to pet owners who aren't sure how to treat these issues. The Colorado State University's Veterinary Teaching Hospital has put some clinical trials in motion to study the effects of CBD on the health of animals.

At this point you might be thinking, *What* doesn't *CBD do?* I have to admit, the ECS seems to be involved in so many physiological processes that it seems harder to find conditions that CBD won't help with than those that it seems to. But as I mentioned before, the ECS is one of the body's largest systems, and its reach extends far and wide. And if you thought we'd covered all of them, you'd be wrong!

It's thought that CBD can counteract the airway hyperactivity and allergic response associated with asthma. Studies have also shown that cannabidiol can speed up the healing process of fractured bones and that cannabinoid receptors trigger bone formation. Studies have been performed on CBD and schizophrenia, CBD and ADHD, and CBD and patients with autism spectrum disorder—which have all produced promising results. There's even reason to suspect that the ECS plays a role in the accumulation of abdominal fat and cardiovascular disease, which makes some sense when you think about THC's ability to trigger hunger and affect blood sugar levels. Studies have shown that factors like meal size, body weight, and even insulin resistance and cholesterol levels can all be affected by the endocannabinoid system.

So is CBD the miracle cure we've all been waiting for? Yes and no. I don't really believe in miracle cures, but I have to admit that CBD has a lot of potential to help a lot of people in a lot of different areas of health, especially those who are currently at the mercy of pharmaceutical drugs that leave a lot to be desired.

6

CBD and Your Skin

Our skin is the largest organ in our body, responsible for protecting us from the outside world—with all its germs, toxins, and other unmentionables—and purging our bodies of impurities through sweating. As with pain, we often take our skin for granted until there's a problem, typically in the form of acne, excessive dryness, an atypical mole, or an inflammatory skin condition like psoriasis. If you start experiencing any of these issues, you'll have to wade through endless prescription and topical products that promise a cure—as long as you pay the hefty price tag and apply all of them, every day, in the correct order. Ugh.

Despite the fact that you can easily spend your entire paycheck on this journey, it turns out that tackling skin issues with excessive products—filled with harsh chemicals, fragrances, and preservatives— might not even be the best approach. We're in the middle of a skin-care revolution, where people are turning away from synthetic products that strip their skin of its natural oils and bacteria and toward ones that are natural, simple, and gentle. You see, skin is a complex ecosystem (it even has its own microbiome!), and therefore if we want to heal it, we might

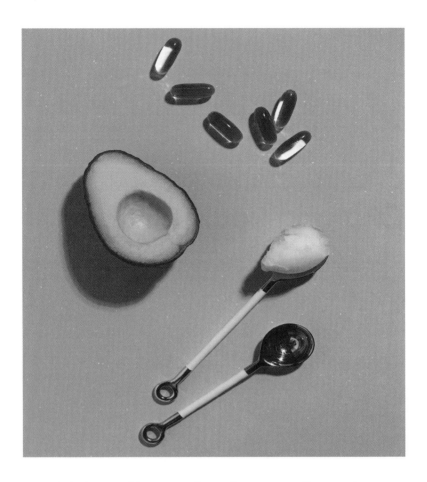

actually be better off leaving it alone. This can actually mean fewer cosmetics and even *less* washing—or only applying products that support the skin's natural bells and whistles like its bacterial balance or antioxidant activity.

This is why when it comes to skin health, CBD has drawn a lot of attention from skin health experts. Its antioxidant properties have made it an attractive ingredient for brands to highlight in antiaging and skin-rejuvenating products, and because of the close relationship between the endocannabinoid system (ECS) and so many other bodily systems—and the fact that some scientists think there may be even more endocannabinoids in the skin than in the brain—experts believe that CBD can support the skin's healthy activity.

CBD AND ANTIOXIDANT SKIN CARE

Just walk through the ground floor of any department store and you'll be practically assaulted by high-antioxidant ingredients like astaxanthin, CoQ10, vitamin C, resveratrol, and vitamin E (the list, quite literally, could go on and on). Why is this? Well, just like the rest of the body, normal aging of the skin can be sped up by factors like too much sun, pollutants, and smoking that produce free radicals in the body. And as I discussed earlier, antioxidants like CBD counteract the damage done by free radicals, which among many things has been linked to premature wrinkles and atypical pigmentation in the skin.

Over the years, studies have shown that the use of topical antioxidants is an effective approach for preventing free radical damage and all that comes with it. Because of CBD's strong antioxidant profile, it's no surprise that beauty and cosmetic companies—especially those that like to take a holistic approach to skin health—have jumped at the opportunity to infuse our beauty routines with CBD. I'm not complaining about this, but when it comes to skin health, CBD shows promise for way more than just wrinkles.

CBD AND INFLAMMATORY SKIN CONDITIONS

The ECS works to regulate cell proliferation, survival, and the immune competence of skin cells. This doesn't mean a lot to most people, so let's just say that disruptions in any of these factors have been connected to acne, allergic dermatitis, itchiness and pain, hair growth disorders, skin cancers, and autoimmune diseases of the skin like eczema and psoriasis. There are a ton of people using topical CBD products in combination with—or, following medical advice, even as a replacement for—their prescription medications. This makes sense, since most of these conditions can be looped into one big category labeled "inflammation of the skin." At this point, a lot of the evidence is anecdotal, but a research report out of the University of Colorado School of Medicine—the first state to legalize weed for recreational use in 2012—did deem both THC and CBD useful for inflammation and itch in cases of psoriasis, eczema, and allergic dermatitis when applied topically to the skin.

CBD AND ACNE

Acne is one of the most common skin conditions around, affecting people ranging from teenagers all the way to women going through menopause. It's currently treated by drugs like antibiotics and Accutane and about 463,839,283,782,293 different kinds of topical products—from retinoids to benzoyl peroxide to charcoal masks—of varying effectiveness. Acne can have a lot of root causes, but one of the main issues is an overproduction of sebum in the sebaceous glands (i.e., your skin is too oily).

As it turns out, the endocannabinoid system is intricately involved in the production of sebum, and CBD has been shown to exhibit sebostatic effects and also helps to reduce inflammation, which is another important factor in acne. Remember when we talked about how the ECS helps regulate the life cycle of our cells? This is also important when it comes to acne. We want to make sure that our skin cells are turning over and being replaced by new, healthier ones. In fact, if you've ever used or heard of retinol, in simple terms, that's basically how it works.

When you're looking for CBD-based skin-care products, there are a few dos and don'ts to keep in mind. The first is to avoid any product that has "fragrance" on the ingredient list—this can mean any number of things and makes a product much more likely to trigger an allergic response. You also want to avoid ingredients like formaldehyde (common in nail polishes), triclosan in soap, and parabens, polyethylene, and phthalates—just to name a few. You'd be shocked to find out how poorly regulated cosmetics are and the nasty ingredients that can end up on your skin and in your hair if you're not discerning. The good news is that there are a ton of resources out there—like the Environmental Working Group—to help you separate the good from the bad, as well as a cornucopia of natural beauty and skin-care lines to lean on. Lucky us!

What's Actually in CBD Oil?

So now you know about the science of CBD and how the endocannabinoid system works, you know a little bit about its history, and you're familiar with some of the conditions it may be able to help with. You might even be ready to try CBD! There are a number of things to know before you start searching for that perfect CBD product—the first of which has everything to do with sourcing. I've already described some of the legal differences between hemp and marijuana, and how CBD oil can be derived from either, but it's not quite that simple. When it comes to making CBD oil (and all herbs, for that matter), the part of the plant used and the way the CBD is extracted from that plant material make all the difference.

DIFFERENT SOURCES OF CBD

For the sake of simplicity, I've decided to categorize CBD oils into roughly three different groups based on what kind of cannabis plant they're made from. Keep in mind that I'm now looking at the difference between hemp and marijuana in terms of health benefits, so for scientific purposes the legal definition matters less than whether or not the plant being used is safe, effective, and contains appropriate levels of CBD to actually do its job in your body.

Industrial Hemp-Derived CBD

Industrialized hemp is the type of hemp many people associate with hippies, clothing, and hempseed oil. Industrial hemp looks, well, industrial. It's tall and has long stalks, it's full of seeds, it's not cultivated to produce buds (also known as the *flowering portion*), and it's most likely imported from Europe or China.

Producing CBD oil from industrialized hemp is the most legal way to do it, but many CBD experts will say it also makes for the lowest-quality product. This is because the cannabinoid content in industrialized hemp is extremely limited. Remember when I talked about how hemp is low in not just THC but all the cannabinoids, including CBD? This is the type of hemp I was specifically referring to. Companies that use industrialized hemp can be applauded for operating aboveboard, but the quality of the product can easily be called into question.

Put simply, this type of hemp is not grown specifically for the flower or oils, and because of this, a lot of plant material is needed to extract useful concentrations of CBD. This is an issue because hemp is a bio-accumulator or phytoremediator, meaning it absorbs heavy metals and chemicals from the soil. The more plant you use, the more likely you are to get higher concentrations of contaminants, which is obviously not good.

All that said, some larger supplement companies are starting to produce hemp oil supplements made from non-GMO, pesticide-free industrialized hemp that has been grown on organic hemp farms and tested rigorously for potency and purity. They don't want to take the legal risk of producing CBD oil from the flowering portions—which is understandable—but still want to create a high-quality product that acts more as a supplement to support the endocannabinoid system as a whole than strictly as a CBD oil.

Therapeutic Hemp-Derived CBD

Somewhere between the stalky, industrialized hemp described above and medical marijuana is a type of hemp that is now known as *therapeutic hemp*. These plants might still look slightly industrial, but they have a higher concentration of CBD, terpenes, and other cannabinoids. Therapeutic hemp is typically grown in the United States in a state that has legalized marijuana for recreation. In many ways, you can think of therapeutic hemp as medical marijuana with the THC bred out so that it qualifies as "hemp" under the Farm Bill of 2014. This might seem far-fetched at first, but there are cannabis plants—like a strain called AC/DC—that *naturally* have CBD-to-THC ratios as high as 35:1.

I recommend looking for a CBD oil derived from therapeutic hemp, as you're more likely to find a product that's rich in cannabinoids and terpenes. An added benefit is that companies using this type of hemp generally know exactly where, how, and when the therapeutic hemp is grown and are in charge of their entire supply chain, from farming to extraction to packaging. Many of the companies getting their hemp from other countries can't say the same.

Even though these companies operate in that legal gray area mentioned earlier—since the Farm Bill is a bit unclear, and they are likely using the entire plant, including the flowering portion—this type of hemp is grown specifically for its medicinal value and oftentimes by farmers who are also growing medical marijuana. In other words, they're pros. The downside here is that technically, at any point, the government could start cracking down on these companies.

Marijuana-Derived CBD

You'll be happy to know that that this section is pretty cut-and-dried, and that's because marijuana-derived CBD is sold only in states with recreational marijuana, where no one is too concerned with the legal difference between hemp and marijuana. Phew, right? I say states with *recreational* marijuana because while it is possible to get CBD oil through a medical marijuana dispensary if you qualify for a medical marijuana card, doing it this way can be insanely expensive, and the products are often extremely limited. (I'm talking one or two options total.) In contrast, states with recreational marijuana have a lot more competition, and therefore, there are a ton of different brands and options to choose from. This is why I personally would stick to the therapeutic hemp-based CBD products that you can get online—unless you're in a state that has legalized cannabis for recreation, and in that case, you can find a dispensary with knowledgeable people to help you.

The products you find in dispensaries are technically made from marijuana, but many of them are nonintoxicating. This is because they are either made from cannabis that is naturally low in THC, as I mentioned before, or the oil has been put through a process that extracts the THC while leaving the other cannabinoids alone. These CBD products will use the flowering portion—since, again, they don't have to worry about the legal definition of "hemp" being only the stalks and seeds. Wouldn't it be nice if all states had this kind of freedom?

THE PERFECT RATIO OF CBD TO THC

When you visit a dispensary and ask for high-CBD products, you unknowingly open a big can of worms. You'll quickly be confronted with CBD-to-THC ratios ranging from around 35:1 to 10:1 to 4:1 all the way to 1:1. Products with a higher ratio of CBD to THC (10:1 or 18:1) are normally recommended for anxiety or general wellness, and many people say that after a little bit of trial and error, they find a ratio that works the best for them. The cutoff point for intoxication is about 8:1 CBD to THC—meaning that anything below that will get you high and anything above that will be nonintoxicating, depending on your specific tolerance.

It's important to remember that, like dosing CBD, finding the perfect ratio of CBD to THC is more of an art than a science. In addition, the ratio that works best for you might change depending on what it is that currently ails you. For example, one ratio might be effective for a migraine and another will work better for a panic attack. Some people report that they don't feel any immediate and noticeable sensation when taking hemp-based CBD products because of the low THC con-

Success Stories: Leigh, Thirty-One

I've struggled with insomnia since I was thirteen years old. For as long as I can remember, I've spent at least two nights a week staring at the ceiling, willing myself to fall asleep as my mind listed off all the things I was worried about on an endless loop, no matter how irrational. By the time I finally I got to sleep, dawn would be breaking and I'd have to wake up just a few hours later. I'd spend the entire day completely exhausted, running on coffee and the little brainpower I had left.

I've tried everything, from meditation and regular exercise to magnesium and prescription drugs. I even tried hemp-based CBD oil, but that didn't seem to do much for me. I recently started eating two Satori cannabis-infused chocolate-covered almonds a few hours before bed, and in addition to this snack satisfying my massive post-dinner sweet tooth, I've never slept so well in my life. Something about that 10:1 CBD-to-THC ratio, which is still below the level of intoxication, just does it for me. And it doesn't hurt that they're absolutely delicious.

While I'm still putting other antianxiety practices into place in an effort to sleep better (no technology allowed in the bedroom, daily exercise, the list goes on), it's nice to know that I've finally found a natural, healthy, and delicious solution that I feel comfortable leaning on. Plus, it helps me stay calm and alert throughout the workday when I'm in need of a productivity boost, which certainly beats reaching for a cupcake and dealing with a subsequent sugar crash. How great is that?

tent, but once they start experimenting with ratios with a little bit more THC—like a 10:1 CBD-to-THC ratio—they notice more immediate and profound benefits while still avoiding any intoxicating effects.

This is a whole new side of CBD that you won't be exposed to unless you're in a state that has legalized cannabis and you can visit a dispensary. Hemp-based products can be effective and are currently accessible to everyone—which is their most important quality—but having the freedom to play with CBD-to-THC ratios takes things to a whole new level and creates so much more potential. And as other states (and hopefully the federal government) start embracing cannabis, this is what the future of CBD oil will look like.

A WORD ON THC-FREE PRODUCTS

Despite all this talk about the "entourage effect" and the way THC and CBD work together, you'll see plenty of CBD oils (from dispensaries and hemp-based CBD products) labeled "THC free." This seems counterintuitive: Who is looking for THC-free products when we know about the entourage effect? Well, despite the symbiotic relationship between THC and CBD, quite a few people are still looking to avoid THC altogether.

This would include people like active military personnel, police officers, or firefighters who want the pain- and PTSD-relieving effects of CBD but are forbidden from using any THC-containing products. Even though taking CBD oil in normal amounts probably won't make you fail a drug test (drug tests screen for higher amounts of THC than you would find in a hemp-based CBD oil), people in certain professions will want to avoid THC altogether. Another great example is for children like Charlotte, whose parents, understandably, don't want them exposed to even the smallest dose of THC due to its intoxicating nature and the potential consequences on the developing brain.

> ### A Quick Chemistry Lesson
> Did you know that the compound found naturally in cannabis is actually called CBDA? In order to make CBD, the plant must go through a process called *decarboxylation*, which occurs when you heat it to a certain temperature during the manufacturing process and the CBDA turns into CBD. THC has to go through the same process, which converts the nonintoxicating precursor THCA to THC. For CBD oil, carboxylation is completed during the manufacturing process, but for marijuana, THCA is successfully decarboxylated to THC when it's smoked, which is why smoking is the most common way to use it.

In conclusion, the THC-to-CBD sweet spot is different for each condition and each person, but finding the one that's right for you will allow you to unleash the true therapeutic potential of cannabis. In the next chapter, I'll suggest one way of going about the experimentation process, but for now, it's time to stick to how your CBD oil is made. And that brings us to the different extraction methods.

DIFFERENT EXTRACTION METHODS

Now you know what type of plant CBD oil is made from, but how do you actually get it out of the plant and into the bottle? This part of the process is called *extraction* and it can mean the difference between a good product and a bad one. This chapter is meant to explain the extraction process, but is not a guide to do it yourself.

Most of the time, extracting compounds from an herb requires the use of a solvent, which is a liquid that you add to the raw plant material to pull out the compounds living inside (it's kind of like making tea). Then, you remove the solvent and *voilà*, you have your by-product that you can then bottle or encapsulate! There are a bunch of different kinds of solvents, and some are safer than others. For instance, butane and hexane are great solvents, but they're also potentially harmful to the body, so you want to avoid them because a little bit of solvent residue can sometimes end up in your product. Luckily, when it comes to CBD, the solvents most frequently used seem to be CO_2 extraction, ethanol, and oil extraction—and they're all good choices.

CO_2 extraction uses pressurized carbon to pull out and isolate the cannabinoids from the plant by passing it through different chambers in a big, very expensive machine. This works because although CO_2 is a gas (and most solvents are liquids), at certain temperatures, it acts as a solvent. CO_2 extraction is also frequently used to make coffee and essential oils. You'll often hear this extraction method touted as the best in the business; the only issue is that CO_2 extraction is intricate and requires a lot of very expensive equipment, which means that these products will likely be more expensive. Many people also say that if it's not done correctly, CO_2 extraction can disrupt the structure of the cannabinoids and terpenes, which is why it's important to make sure you're getting your CBD from someone who knows what they're doing.

Ethanol extraction is another common method, and it involves adding ethanol to the plant to draw out the cannabinoids. Ethanol is generally regarded as safe and is commonly used as a preservative in food, so even if a little bit is left behind after the solvent is removed, it's not considered dangerous. The downside of ethanol extraction is that along with the desired terpenes and cannabinoids, other parts of the plant like chlorophyll are also extracted. Some argue that chlorophyll—which is actually the compound that gives plants their green color—is a beneficial substance and contributes to the entourage effect. Others say it's best to avoid chlorophyll in CBD because it makes your CBD oil taste bad. This is definitely a factor if you're taking CBD on its own under your tongue, but for the most part, this book uses flavored CBD in different recipes, and that should mask most of the muskiness from the presence of chlorophyll.

Last but not least, there's lipid extraction, which is typically done using olive oil. With this method, the plant is basically steeped in oil, which draws out the cannabinoids like a big cup of hemp tea. Because of its simplicity, this is a commonly used at-home extraction method. The benefit of oil extraction is that there's a lot less processing overall, since the method of extraction is the form of the final product. The downside? It's highly perishable, so you want to make sure the manufacturer is aware of this and that you're always storing lipid-extracted CBD oil in a cool, dry place. Otherwise, it can turn rancid.

Keep in mind that every CBD company you talk to will boisterously inform you that they are using the number one, safest, most effective extraction method in the world. Obviously, they can't all be right. But there's also no way to really tell which one is the best at this point, with the exception of knowing that butane and hexane are unfavorable. Plus, as a consumer, I'm more concerned with the quality of the finished product. Therefore, as long as the company is testing their final product to make sure all the cannabinoids are intact and there isn't any solvent residue, I don't think you need to rule out any extraction methods completely.

Finding the Right CBD Product for You

There are a number of things to know before you go shopping for CBD products. This chapter outlines what I consider to be the main ones. On this list are the difference between full-spectrum products and isolates, the pros and cons of sublingual oils and edibles, and what questions to ask your CBD company about quality control. Why do you need to know all this? To put it simply: Not all CBD is created equal. And in such a new and developing industry, it largely up to us—the consumers—to separate the good from the bad.

FULL-SPECTRUM HEMP PRODUCTS

When you first start your search for a CBD oil, you'll see a lot of products labeled "full-spectrum." This means that instead of being pure or isolated CBD, the product contains additional cannabinoids and other plant compounds like flavonoids and terpenes, which are basically the essential oils of plants, giving them smell, color, and taste. Keeping these compounds around is important because the entourage effect doesn't just apply to THC and CBD; it applies to *all* the ingredients

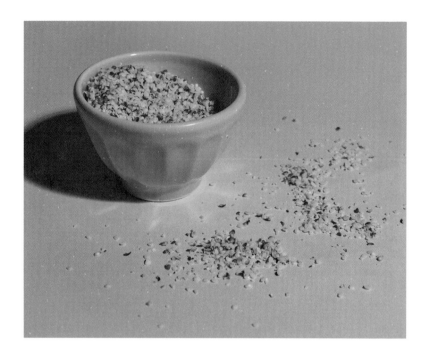

found in the cannabis plant. When you use a full-spectrum hemp oil, you also get the health benefits from these compounds—plus other vitamins, minerals, proteins, and fatty acids that are found in the cannabis plant, too. This is an important point: Hemp oil isn't healthy just because of the CBD; CBD is just an important part of the overall equation. Even hemp seeds are a rich source of essential fatty acids, protein, and vitamin E, which is why they're featured in more than one of the recipes later on.

Almost every CBD expert will tell you that full-spectrum products are the best way to take CBD—or any cannabinoid, for that matter. In fact, some cannabis experts even say that they're just as excited about the potential healing benefits of the terpenes in the plant as the cannabinoids themselves. Research has shown not only that full-spectrum hemp products are more effective but that patients generally prefer the feeling gained from consuming full-spectrum products over synthetic and isolated cannabinoids.

CBD Isolates

CBD isolates are made by isolating CBD and then refining it to a highly potent single-compound product, which gives you an almost pure dose of CBD (about 99 percent). CBD isolates are mostly found in a crystalline form that is more or less tasteless, and they are sometimes used for cooking or to make other CBD products, although they aren't that easy to find, even at dispensaries.

A pure dose of CBD sounds great in theory, but as I mentioned above, these isolates miss out on the entourage effect provided by other plant compounds, and now researchers know that they can also be problematic when it comes to dosing. Without the other cannabinoids to balance it out, pure CBD has a much more narrow therapeutic window, meaning you have to use a *very* specific dose to get the effect you want. This is very different from full-spectrum CBD, which has a wide therapeutic window because of the presence of all the other cannabinoids.

And so, unless you're working with a doctor to tackle a very specific condition and your doctor recommends a CBD isolate,

A Word on Plant Medicine

When we're comparing and contrasting CBD isolates and full-spectrum hemp products, it's worth mentioning that a big part of plant medicine involves forging a connection with the plant itself. Herbalists think that understanding the plant—and information like where it's grown and what it looks and smells like—can help it work more effectively in the body.

It might be strange to think about, but when pharmaceutical companies create a drug, even when it's derived from a plant, they isolate one compound from the rest of the plant or create an entirely synthetic version. This leaves us with a tasteless (unless it's coated in sugar), colorless (unless it's dyed with artificial colors), odorless pill. It also leaves us pretty disconnected with the origin of the remedy—the plant—which has its own natural flavor, coloring, and smell. This is pretty unavoidable in the case of pharmaceutical drugs, but when it comes to alternative medicine, herbs, and CBD, we can try to keep the whole plant together, get to know it, and connect with nature a little more than we're used to.

stick with the full-spectrum CBD oils. They're simple, normally cheaper, and the fact that they're easier to dose renders them more effective for the general public. As it says in the scientific paper published in *Medical Hypotheses* titled "A Tale of Two Cannabinoids": "Numerous cannabis compounds have medicinal attributes, but the therapeutic impact of whole plant cannabis is greater than the sum of its parts."

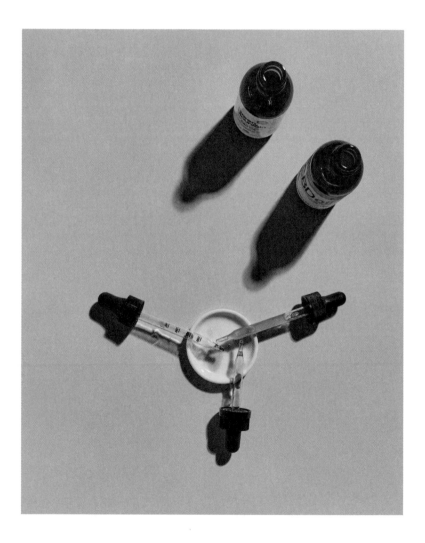

YOUR GUIDE TO DIFFERENT CBD DELIVERY METHODS

Despite the fact that this book is titled *CBD Oil*, there are actually a lot of different ways to take CBD. By this, I mean different delivery methods, like sublingual oils and vape pens and edibles and even transdermal patches. So let's dive in and learn why when it comes to CBD, oil is really just the beginning.

Sublingual Oils and Sprays

Sublingual oils are by far the most popular way to take CBD. These small tincture bottles are versatile and straightforward, and the cannabidiol is normally diluted in a healthy oil like olive oil or coconut oil, which helps it get absorbed into the body. You take these sublingual oils by simply dropping the correct dose under your tongue, waiting about sixty seconds, and then swallowing it. Many people report feeling the effects right away, but the general rule is to wait about twenty minutes before you make any conclusions. You can also find products that you spray under your tongue, and these tend to be easier to dose than a tincture bottle.

Using CBD this way is quick and easy if you're looking for fast relief, but it's also a little bit boring. I'd rather make taking CBD a daily ritual that really forces me to slow down, like in the case of a CBD-infused bath bomb, or savor the taste of whatever CBD-infused treat I'm cooking up. If you do go for the quick and dirty under-the-tongue method, make sure you check out the "other ingredients in your CBD oil" section, since you can buy CBD infused with flavors like vanilla oil and turmeric to make this method a little bit sweeter.

Edibles

The second most common way to take CBD is through food and drink. There is some overlap here with sublingual oils, because as regular consumers—and not big CBD manufacturers who would probably use a more raw form of CBD to make their prepackaged edibles—we use sublingual oils to infuse our food and drink. CBD oils based in coconut oil or olive oil can easily be added to your food or drinks, or used to make any number of recipes in this book.

When you put CBD in your food or drink, it has to be broken down by your digestive system, and that takes time. This is why edibles are considered the slowest delivery method for CBD. That being said, it's also the delivery method that lasts the longest. Therefore, if you're looking for all-day stress relief or longstanding anti-inflammatory effects, CBD-infused chocolates or smoothies are great options. It's less likely that you'll notice any profound changes in how you feel when you take CBD through food because of the gentle, slow absorption and

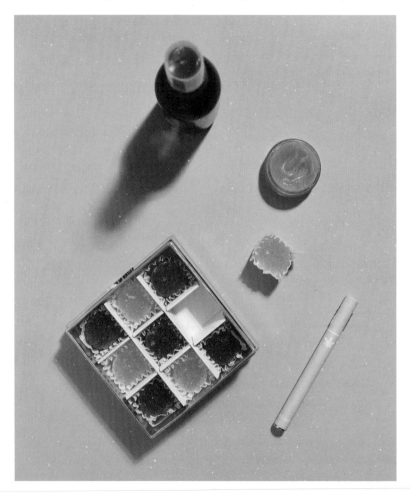

long-lasting effects, but it's a great delivery method for everyday health and wellness and to take consistently over time.

A quick note here: If you decide to experiment with different ratios of CBD to THC, do *not* do it with edibles. I repeat, do *not* do it with edibles. THC tends to be stronger when it's broken down in the digestive system, and it can be hours before it takes effect, which causes a lot of people to double up their dose, only to regret it an hour or two later.

Capsules

It feels like there are more ways to take CBD every single day—a lot of brands are starting to come out with supplement capsules. This is a quick and convenient option, but as with sublingual oils, it takes a lot of the ritual out of using CBD oil and can leave you disconnected from the fact that you're using a natural remedy at all. Plus, who would want to take a pill when they could make a CBD-infused snack? Like edibles, capsules provide a slower release of CBD because they have to be absorbed through your digestive tract. I'd recommend an oil over a capsule because it's just one less barrier the CBD has to get through to get absorbed into your body. That being said, it might be great if you're traveling or going through a particularly stressful time and you just don't have time to think about it.

Topical Products

CBD is also available in the form of topical creams, ointments, soaps, and even bath salts. There's some debate about whether or not these topical products actually absorb into the bloodstream, and you'll hear a lot of conflicting information about it. This debate seems silly to me, since the only real reason to use a topical product is for a topical issue (say, to heal a bug bite or to give your skin an antioxidant boost). And since there aren't any known risks with taking CBD orally, you should be able to choose between capsules, oils, or edibles without a problem if you have a concern that is more than skin deep.

If the issue you're struggling with is something like knee pain or joint stiffness, subject to medical advice, you might try experimenting with both topical and oral delivery methods to see what brings you the most relief. If you're looking to address an internal issue but can't take oral CBD for some reason, a few different companies have transdermal patches that use a special delivery method to make sure the cannabinoids get all the way through the skin and into the bloodstream.

Vaporizers

When I learned that people are vaping CBD, it gave me pause, since puffing on a vape pen isn't exactly the picture of wellness, but I still think they're worth learning about. A vaporizer heats and releases CBD oil in a fine mist that you then inhale. There is no combustion, so many people think that vaping is much safer than smoking because you avoid some of the toxins, carcinogens, and chemicals released when the plant material is burned. But the reality is that we still don't really know what the risks of taking CBD this way might be.

I'm mentioning vaporizers because although there are questions about their safety, many people use them to experiment with different ratios of CBD to THC. This is because they are widely considered one of the faster delivery methods, so theoretically, a person would be able to see how they reacted to a ratio more quickly than with a sublingual oil or an edible. This might be a selling point for some people, but for others, that might not justify the potential risks. At the end of the day, it's up to you to weigh the pros and cons of vape pens if you're interested in taking CBD in this way.

WHAT YOU NEED TO KNOW ABOUT QUALITY CONTROL

I have explained how CBD laws and regulations are a bit of a mess, so naturally, when you're searching for the right CBD oil, you have to spend some time learning how to pick a product that's safe and high quality. This is easier said than done. As mentioned earlier, CBD products are not subject to good manufacturing practices, which is a system that ensures that products are made according to specific quality standards. This means that there isn't any type of larger agency making sure that what's on the label of your CBD oil is actually in the bottle.

Remember how the Food and Drug Administration investigated

CBD companies in 2015? Well, when they tested a bunch of CBD oil in a lab, they found that quite a few products didn't contain as much CBD as it said on the bottle—and some didn't contain any CBD at all. Unfortunately, the lack of regulation does leave you vulnerable to wasting a lot of money and missing out on the true benefits of CBD. This section is all about empowering yourself as a consumer to hopefully minimize the chances of your getting stuck with one of those crappy products.

So far, I've talked about quality in terms of the type of cannabis plant used. And while this is definitely still an important factor, I also have to zoom out and note that farming practices, manufacturing protocols, and even packaging matter a lot when it comes to quality. Because of the lack of good manufacturing practices, it's up to you to ask questions about the whole process so you can make an informed choice when you're looking to start taking CBD.

I know it feels like a lot to take on, but the more informed you are, the easier it will be to experiment. Below is a series of questions you should be able to answer about a CBD oil before you buy.

For now, remember that the idea here is simple: If you call, email, message, or meet the company, they should know the answers to these questions—at a basic level, at least.

1. Is each bottle tested for potency? In other words, if a CBD oil says there are 500 mg in the bottle, are there actually 500 mg of CBD in the bottle?

2. Does every batch go through rigorous testing for contamination? This includes heavy metals, microbes (like bacteria and mold), leftover solvents, and pesticides. Remember, hemp is a bioaccumulator, and that means the company needs to be extremely diligent about testing for heavy metal and chemical contamination at different stages in the manufacturing process.

3. Are all these tests done by a third-party, accredited lab? Can they show you a certificate of analysis? Go ahead and grill your CBD company about this paperwork, which will show you the chemical

composition of the oil and also that it is free from contaminants. They might not be able to tell you the exact lab they use (since some are under a confidentiality agreement), but they should be able to tell you that they do third-party testing from an accredited lab that follows procedures certified by the International Organization for Standardization (ISO). If they don't know what any of that means, it's a red flag.

4. Are they in charge of their entire supply chain? In other words: Does the company grow the cannabis, extract the CBD, and then bottle it themselves? It's a good sign if a company is in control of, or at least very familiar with, the whole process, from harvest to bottle. If not, can they tell you about the farm where it's grown? Do they know a little bit or a lot about the farming practices used? (Hint: They should know a lot.)

5. Are they in charge of premarket and postmarket procedures? If the answer is yes, it means there are procedures in place to address adverse event reporting. In other words, if there's a problem with one of their products, there's a place to report it and a team that will address it.

This is the ideal wish list, and not every company—especially smaller ones—will be able to meet all of these standards. But if you call them or inquire on their website, they should be more than willing to produce lab tests and explain their quality control procedures *in detail*. If they dodge you or have no details to share, picture the operation as one person growing hemp in his backyard and extracting the CBD in his bathtub (yes, this does happen), and move on to a company that's more transparent.

OTHER INGREDIENTS HIDING IN YOUR CBD

During your search for the perfect CBD oil, you might encounter some unexpected ingredients in the products you consider. When it comes to sublingual oils and tinctures, the base will most likely be coconut oil, olive oil, or something called MCT oil. MCT stands for medium-chain triglycerides, and these fats make up about 60 percent of the total fat content in coconut oil. MCTs are praised for their ability to support the metabolism, heart, and healthy cognition and energy levels.

If you're knee-deep in CBD products, you've also probably encountered ingredients like turmeric, orange, or mint. These ingredients provide an additional nutrient boost, and they also give the oil a different flavor profile. Turmeric, for example, is praised for its anti-inflammatory properties, and a little bit of natural orange flavor really completes my CBD-Infused After-Dinner Drink (page 147).

> ## Avoiding Unhealthy Fats
> I have yet to encounter a CBD oil product with these ingredients, but just to cover all the bases, remember to avoid anything made with oils like corn oil, peanut oil, palm oil, or hydrogenated oils. And this rule doesn't just apply to CBD. Some fats (like those found in avocados and olive oil) are inflammation-fighting superfoods, and others—like the hydrogenated oils found in common peanut butters and margarine—can actually trigger inflammation and wreak havoc on your body. Not all fats are created equal, and one of the best nutrition skills you can possess is the ability to differentiate good fats from bad fats right on the spot.

The way unflavored CBD oil tastes depends on a lot of different factors, especially the extraction method used and how the company processes the CBD after that. Some oils taste pretty mild, and others taste, well, let's call it *earthy*. It can take some trial and error to figure out which brands and products you enjoy; some people prefer the milder products, and others like to celebrate the natural flavors of the plant. The good news is that there's a lot of diversity. You'll find that I sometimes recommend a specific flavor for a recipe—cue the lovely Mint Chip Afternoon Smoothie (page 119) infused with chocolate-mint-flavored CBD oil from a company in Vermont—and that's to highlight how creative brands are starting to get with their formulations.

Last but not least, remember that when you're reading ingredients, you want to avoid any artificial food dyes, synthetic flavors, or unnecessary preservatives. As a general rule, the "additional ingredients" section on the label should be as short as possible. If you see a bunch of ingredients you don't recognize or can't pronounce, that's a warning sign that a lot of things have been added to and subtracted from the oil, which is likely a hint that the original product wasn't of the highest quality.

WHERE TO BUY YOUR CBD

I've talked a lot about what increases your chances of finding a great CBD product. But where do you buy it? You have a few options here. You can buy hemp-based CBD products in some health food stores and online, and if you live in a state with recreational marijuana, you can buy your CBD oil at a dispensary as long as you're twenty-one years old.

A Buyer's Checklist to Hemp-Based CBD Products

If you're looking to buy a hemp-based CBD oil, you'll likely be confronted with a lot of options. This is true in health food stores, but it's even more applicable on the Internet. I've already described some of the key characteristics of what makes a good product, so let's just recap. Here's your CBD-buying checklist.

- Ideally, look for CBD oil from organic, non-GMO, CBD-rich hemp. As an aside, under current law you cannot call any marijuana "organic," so if you're getting your CBD at a dispensary, you won't find any organic products, but you can still grill the manufacturer about their farming practices and whether or not they use pesticides.
- Choose a full-spectrum hemp product over a THC-free product or a CBD isolate, unless you have a specific reason to seek those products out.
- Ideally, buy a product extracted from the entire plant, including the flowering portion, which is the part with the significant cannabinoid content.

- Look for a brand that has been third-party lab tested for contaminants (like mold, bacteria, and heavy metals) and potency by an accredited lab that is making sure the products meet all standards for purity, potency, and safety. Look for a batch number on the label or packaging.
- Find a CBD oil based in a healthy fat like olive oil or MCT oil.
- Avoid any added ingredients that don't contribute to the therapeutic value of the CBD; this includes things like artificial colors, flavors, fillers, or preservatives.

Remember, not all brands will meet every single one of these standards to perfection. That doesn't mean they're garbage, but it's up to you to weigh the pros and cons and conduct a cost-benefit analysis. Just remember, you're taking CBD for your health, and you deserve the highest-quality ingredients available for the price you can afford! In this recipe section, I included some brands that I have tried and enjoyed, and like to add to specific recipes because of their flavor profiles.

How to Get CBD from a Dispensary

If you live in a state with recreational marijuana or have a medical marijuana card, you might want to try getting your CBD oil from a dispensary. If you do this, proceed with caution. The big lessons I learned visiting dispensaries were that a) the CBD products were extremely popular and oftentimes completely sold out, and b) it can be really difficult to figure out what to buy and how to take it.

Does that second one surprise you? It shocked me, too. My expectations were high when I first went to a dispensary, and I was hoping to be gently ushered to the CBD products, where I would gain answers to all my most pressing questions and confusions. Instead, I talked to a number of different people who gave me a lot of conflicting information and handed me a bunch of products that were poorly labeled. For the cherry on top, many of the companies are still very secretive about their sourcing, so it's hard to get the answers you're looking for. I quickly figured out that not all products in dispensaries are high quality.

Many people will say this is overly harsh, so let me explain exactly what I mean. Some products will say "high CBD" but not tell you if there's any THC in them or if they are intoxicating or not. I was pretty flabbergasted that some products would just say something like "CBD vape pen" and then not give any more information. If you conduct an online search to find out more about a product, you might not even be able to find a website.

And so the best rule I can give you is this: If you're getting your CBD from a dispensary, look for products that are explicitly labeled "nonintoxicating," and look for a brand that provides answers to all your questions right on the packaging. I also recommend going to a dispensary where they require you to have a one-on-one consultation, so you're not running around trying to pin someone down like you're at the Apple store looking for help from the Genius bar.

Legal cannabis in the United States is a young, budding (pun intended) industry, but the question is pretty simple: Should I really know more about what's in my granola bar than my CBD oil? In my opinion, when it comes to the products that leave you with more questions than answers—don't even give them a second glance. Be cutthroat about this. You shouldn't have to play any guessing games with your health and well-being.

Taking CBD for the First Time

You've read about the history, science, and healing potential of CBD. You've learned how it's grown, extracted, and made. You've sought medical advice and done your research. You've found the perfect CBD oil that meets all your standards for quality and taste. You're ready to take it for a spin!

If you're at this stage, you might find that dosing CBD is a little more complicated than you thought. And even though each product has dosing instructions, they can vary, and there's not much info out there telling you what dose to use for specific concerns. For instance: Which dose is best for migraines? And what about sleep? In this chapter, we'll cover some approaches to answering these questions.

Before we start, it's important to know that you should always talk to your doctor before starting any new supplement—especially if you have a chronic health issue or are on medication of any kind. I don't want to sound like a broken record, but there's still a lot researchers don't know about CBD and how it interacts with the body. Always err on the side of caution, and if you have a great doctor, he or she might even do some research for you or talk to colleagues who have prescribed CBD to give you some guidance. Alternatively, consulting a health care professional who is well versed in cannabis science can make this whole dosing process a lot easier. This expert can help you decide exactly what dose and delivery method is right for you and your health concerns.

That being said, consultations can be hard to find and are often expensive, so many of us end up simply informing our doctors that we're going to try CBD—and then going it alone.

I know you're hoping for a really simple answer to the question, How much CBD should I take? Unfortunately, this one doesn't come with a simple answer. Because of CBD's diverse nature, the way CBD isolate reacts differently in the body from a full-spectrum hemp oil, and the fact that everyone reacts to cannabinoids in a unique way, dosing is all over the place. For example, doses for CBD-derived pharmaceutical drugs range anywhere from 2.5 mg (this is a drug with equal parts CBD and THC) to about 1,400 mg (for pure CBD isolate). Clearly, this is a *big* difference and requires some further explanation. To start, we need to address the biphasic nature of CBD.

THE BIPHASIC NATURE OF CBD

To be *biphasic* is to have differing effects on the body at different concentrations. Practically speaking, this means that a drug will have one effect at one dose and the opposite effect at others. Alcohol is a perfect example of a biphasic substance that anyone who's had a few too many drinks is familiar with: It's a stimulant until a certain point, and then it quickly becomes a depressant.

CBD is biphasic as well, and this explains why dosing can be confusing and why sometimes you'll hear conflicting information about its health benefits. Insomnia is the perfect example; you might hear that CBD is great for sleep, and then a few seconds later someone will praise it for its energizing effects and ability to increase alertness. The truth is that CBD has been shown to do both of those things—just at different doses. This also means that doubling your dose of CBD won't make it twice as strong; in fact, it might actually render it less effective.

You might be thinking, *That's all well and good, Gretchen, but where the hell I am supposed to start?* For CBD-rich hemp extracts, most experts recommend starting with doses as low as 3 or 5 mg and then titrating up from there. An important thing to remember is that the best dose of CBD for you doesn't have much to do with how much you weigh or whether you're a man or women, like so many other drugs. Instead, it has everything to do with how your cannabinoid receptors are clustered in your body and the current status of your ECS tone, which is one of the reasons why there are no official recommendations when it comes to CBD dosage.

What does this look like in real life? Well, one person's headache might respond to 6 mg of CBD, while another person with the same type of headache might need 50 mg. There's also quite a bit of intrapersonal variation, which means that one day you might need twice as much as you did the day before. The good news is that full-spectrum hemp products have a really good safety profile, so it's okay to play around.

THE BEGINNER'S GUIDE TO DOSING CBD

The dosing conversation can be overwhelming, and it makes a lot of people nervous. Please don't worry—there haven't been any reports of someone having a violent reaction from taking the wrong dose of CBD. Its effects are pretty subtle! The key is to start low, remember that less is more, and always stay in tune with your body.

As I mentioned before, there are no official recommendations for dosing CBD, but based on clinical observation and patient testimonials, most people are taking between 10 and 100 mg daily. Most CBD products are dosed at about 15 mg twice a day, so 30 mg seems to be the average daily dose. First make sure that you have spoken to a health care professional to make sure that there is no reason that you shouldn't be experimenting with CBD, especially if you are pregnant, taking medication, or have any kind of medical condition. Once that is done, here are some suggestions:

1. Start with about 5 mg twice daily for a few days.

2. If you don't feel any change, try moving up to 10 mg twice daily.

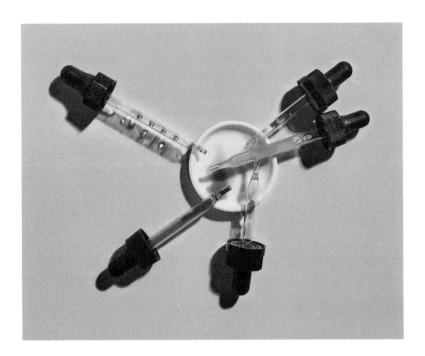

3. Continue titrating up, waiting a few days before increasing the dose, all the way up to 45 mg twice a day. Stay here consistently for a few weeks to a few months—many people say it takes that much time to reach the full potential.

4. If you're thinking about going higher, this is a good place to pause and consult a professional if you haven't already. Over 100 mg is considered a "high dose" of CBD.

You might notice a difference when you take CBD with food, on an empty stomach, or with a liquid versus a food. That's normal, as whatever is in your stomach can affect the absorption rate. Just keep paying attention to how you feel. While you're going through this process of experimenting with CBD, it's a great idea to keep a journal or log your symptoms on your calendar.

Some CBD Safety Questions—Answered

As I've mentioned, the safety profile of CBD is pretty miraculous. But what does this really mean? I talked to a lot of CBD experts while writing this book, and every single one said that at normal doses (this is generally considered under 100 mg of CBD a day) there are no big safety concerns like overdosing and CBD-drug interactions. To date and according to research, taking higher doses of CBD has been associated with symptoms like headaches and fatigue, but so far nothing more serious than that.

That being said, it's definitely worth mentioning that at certain levels, CBD has been shown to temporarily deactivate cytochrome P450, which is an important group of enzymes that work to metabolize a wide range of drugs and compounds that enter the body. You've probably heard the rule that you shouldn't eat grapefruit with certain medications, and that's because grapefruit also blocks cytochrome P450. Unfortunately, there is no exact cutoff dose for CBD and its interaction with P450, so the best game plan is that if you are taking CBD long-term or at higher doses and are on any other medications, talk to a doctor.

Experimenting with CBD-to-THC Ratios

If you're lucky enough to live in a state that has legalized recreational marijuana, you might want to try inching up the THC levels in your CBD oil. But where do you start? After much experimentation and trial and error—and multiple THC-induced panic attacks suffered by me and one of my dear friends who was happy to act as guinea pig for my research—this is one strategy for going about experimenting with different ratios of CBD to THC. Keep in mind that it's subject to your experience with and reactions to THC and its legality in your state.

Start with the highest ratio of CBD to THC you can find, especially if you've had a negative reaction to THC in the past. Normally, this is a 30:1, 20:1, or 18:1 ratio, and I would recommend beginning with a sublingual oil, spray, or vape pen delivery method, as these will work faster so you can observe the effects right away.

Once you have your first product, take half of the recommended dose. Wait about thirty minutes to see how you feel, and then try going up to the full recommended dose. If you get the desired effects, feel free to stop there and continue using that dose and that ratio. If you're ready to try the next ratio, don't go from 18:1 to 2:1. Try something more like 10:1, and do the same thing where you try half a dose and observe what happens, then continue down the line until you find the best dose and ratio for you. And remember: Once you get below 8:1, you may start to feel some of the intoxicating effects of THC.

So, you've tracked down a great CBD oil—either from a dispensary or online—and you're ready to give it a try. What can you expect to feel? A lot of people describe feeling centered, calmer, and "relaxed but not intoxicated." Research is suggesting that CBD might have immediate antidepressant effects, so pay attention to any small changes in mood you experience. It's very likely that you'll feel CBD's effects the first time you try it, but like a lot of other herbs, you might want to give it a few weeks of taking it consistently to achieve the results you're looking for.

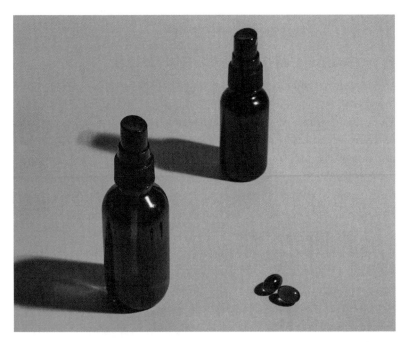

CBD in the Kitchen: Twenty Recipes for Daily Wellness

And now, the moment we've been waiting for. This is where the real fun begins! It's time to bring CBD into the kitchen. On the following pages, you'll find easy recipes that will help you incorporate CBD into your day—some of which might improve your diet, up your antioxidant intake, help fight inflammation, and create a few minutes for yourself at the same time. As I mentioned earlier, improving your health and preventing illness is about way more than just CBD. Keep in mind that these recipes were designed for adults and that it's always important to talk to a healthcare professional before adding anything new to your wellness regime. This is especially true if you are pregnant, breastfeeding, taking a medication, or if you have a chronic health issue.

Embracing an Antioxidant-Rich, Anti-Inflammatory Diet

Every single one of these recipes was created with a different aspect of your health—and a specific benefit of CBD—in mind. For example, rosemary is well-known for improving memory and cognition, and therefore the Rosemary Toasted Nuts (page 141) make the perfect

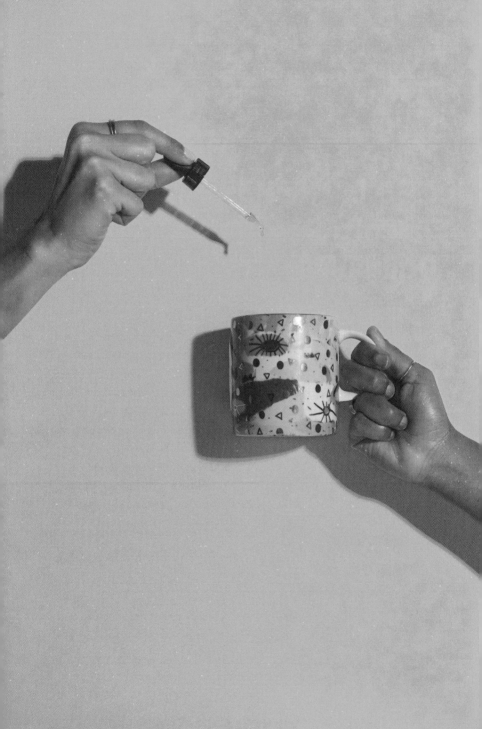

brain-healthy late-night study snack. Turmeric is another super-potent anti-inflammatory ingredient, so the Supergood Golden Milk (page 111) is all about fighting inflammation.

The recipes are largely dairy-free, and although you'll see a few dates or a little bit of maple syrup from time to time, they are very low in sugar—since as previously noted, both dairy and sugar (among other foods) can contribute to inflammation in the body. The inspiration for these recipes was simple: I wanted them to be healthy *and* fun. Too often those concepts feel mutually exclusive.

You'll see a lot of healthy fats featured here, and they're included for more than just their inflammation-fighting properties. Cannabinoids are fat-soluble, which means they break down and are stored well in fat. It also means that taking CBD with fats—like coconut oil, cashew butter, chia seeds, olive oil, hemp seeds, or avocado—will help it get absorbed into the body more efficiently. Remember when I talked about how endocannabinoids are created from essential fatty acids in the body? Well, researchers suspect that omega-3s influence endocannabinoids and activate endocannabinoid receptors, and that a deficiency in omega-3s sabotages endocannabinoid system function. In other words, if you're not getting enough omega-3s, your CBD won't work as well as it should.

You can find most of the required ingredients at any standard grocery store, but some of the recipes include an "optional superfood boost," which features an ingredient that you'll probably have to get at a health food store or online. This optional boost will add some extra healing power to the recipe, but also add to the price tag—which is why it's optional! All of the recipes will work with neutral-flavored CBD oil, but at times I'll suggest specific products with fun flavors as well, in case you feel like mixing it up.

Dosing and Other Nitty-Gritty Details

I've already discussed CBD dosing and how confusing it can be, so how are you supposed to dose CBD for these recipes? Before you start baking and blending and boiling, I'd recommend experimenting with different doses under your tongue. When you find the dose that works for you, use that amount for each serving in the following recipes. If you don't feel like experimenting or just can't feel a noticeable change between different doses of CBD, go ahead and follow the directions on the bottle, which is typically about 15 mg of hemp-based CBD oil, a single dose. When it comes to the beauty and self-care recipes, sometimes you'll be using a balm or topical oil, and these are harder to measure. Don't stress—you're getting CBD on your skin, and that's what really matters.

Calling all mathematicians! I am not one. In fact, just the memory of having to pass college calculus makes my stomach hurt. Nonetheless, sometimes figuring out how much CBD to use can require a few numbers and conversions. Here's what I mean: CBD is best measured in milligrams, but sometimes CBD oils will be dosed in milliliters. If this is the case, make sure you look to see how many *milligrams* of CBD are in each *milliliter* of oil. This might feel complicated, but it comes down to this simple fact: You can't assume that 1 mL of one type of CBD oil will provide the same amount of CBD as the next. For example, two drops of a high-potency oil could provide 15 mg of CBD, but it could take a full dropperful to get 15 mg in a lower-potency oil.

This doesn't have to do with the quality of the product; it has to do with the size of the bottle and how concentrated the company decided to make the oil. As a rule, the label should always tell you how many milligrams of CBD are in each serving size and how many milligrams are in the entire bottle. If your mind just exploded, my best advice is to go grab your friends who like math and force them to help you.

You'll also notice that CBD is often added to the recipe at the end. This is because at this point, CBD chefs aren't sure exactly how much CBD can be heated before it denatures or becomes less effective. Some people say it can be heated without a problem, and others say it shouldn't be heated above a certain temperature. If one of the recipes requires you to heat something on the stove or in the oven, add the CBD after it's taken off the heat, just to be safe.

It might take a little bit of practice to get the dosing and order of operations correct, but once you do, the recipes on the following pages are designed to be fun, delicious, and easy to make. They are filled with antioxidants, anti-inflammatory superfoods, and gut- and brain-supporting nutrients that beautifully complement the healing properties of CBD that you just learned about. Feel free to pick and choose, make them all, and share them with your friends.

One last thing before we get started: For some of the recipes, like the Chocolate-Raspberry Mousse (page 129) and the Cookie Dough Bites (page 127), you'll definitely need a high-speed blender and a food processor, respectively. When it comes to blenders, I really do recommend investing in a Vitamix if you can swing it. I know, it feels insane to spend that kind of money on a blender, but it really does make healthy living a *lot* easier, and you just won't get the same amazingly smooth consistency with other blenders. Expert tip: Vitamix sells refurbished products online that are good as new and have a much lower price tag.

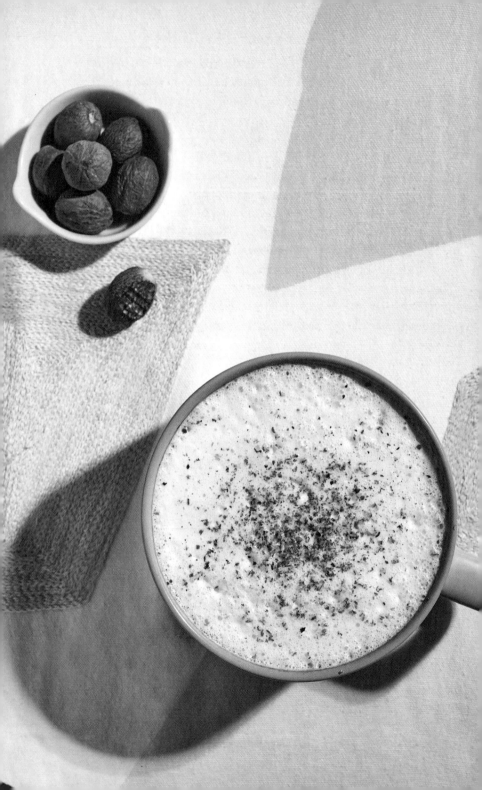

TEAS, TONICS, AND SMOOTHIES

CBD Oil London Fog

I discovered London Fogs about five years ago, and since then, I've taken it upon myself to tell everyone—especially baristas—all about them and how freaking great they are. They combine the gentle caffeine boost of black tea with the sweet, creamy deliciousness of vanilla and steamed milk. They are perfect for winter mornings or a cozy afternoon work session. By adding CBD, you get anti-inflammatory, antioxidant, and anti-anxiety benefits (this one helps me start my day off right).

SERVES 1

Ingredients

1½ cups unsweetened nondairy milk (I'm obsessed with Elmhurst plant-based nut milks, especially the hazelnut)

¼ teaspoon vanilla extract

⅛ teaspoon Ceylon cinnamon

1 bag Earl Grey tea (or substitute noncaffeinated rooibos)

½ teaspoon honey

1 dose (about 15 mg) neutral- or vanilla-flavored CBD oil

Optional superfood boost: 1 teaspoon MCT oil (I like Bulletproof Brain Octane Oil)

Pinch of nutmeg, for garnish

Method

1. Heat milk, vanilla, and cinnamon in a small saucepan, stirring occasionally until a little bit of steam is rising.
2. Turn off the heat and steep tea in the saucepan with the lid on for approximately 5 minutes (a little longer if you like your tea really strong).
3. Remove the tea bag and empty the warm milk into a blender, adding the honey, CBD oil, and optional MCT oil.
4. Blend on high until the mixture is nice and frothy on top.
5. Pour the tea (including all the foam!) into your biggest mug.
6. Add a pinch of nutmeg for a cozy and luxurious drink. Serve immediately.

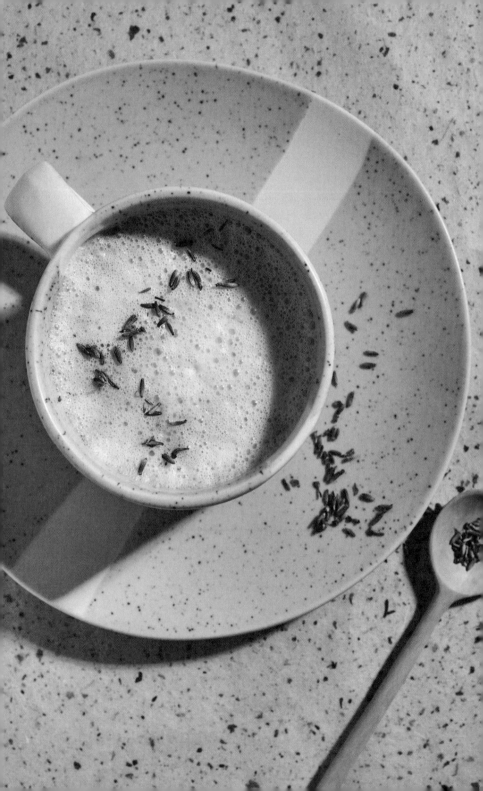

Lavender Latte

There's something beautiful about combining the stimulating nature of coffee with the world-famous calming properties of lavender. Adding CBD to the mix brings in some extra relaxing properties, perfect for people who are sensitive to caffeine but have a hard time breaking up with coffee. (I'm definitely on this list.) This latte is just sweet enough, and the aroma of lavender is there, but it's not overwhelming. If you're a big fan, make a quadruple batch of lavender syrup and keep some in the fridge for quick and easy lavender lattes all week.

SERVES 1

Lavender Simple Syrup Ingredients

½ cup water

1 tablespoon dried lavender (you can get this at most specialty tea shops)

1 teaspoon coconut sugar

¼ teaspoon vanilla extract

Latte Ingredients

2 ounces espresso (about 2 shots) or extra-strong coffee (dark or Italian roast)

1 dose (about 15 mg) of your favorite CBD oil (I like Juna's Nude CBD oil)

6 ounces nondairy barista milk (I like New Barn Barista Almondmilk)

Method

1. Add the water, lavender, sugar, and vanilla to a small saucepan, and heat just to a boil. Reduce heat and simmer with the lid on to preserve the lavender essential oils for 5 to 7 minutes.

continued

2. Pour the infusion through a strainer to remove the dried lavender, into your mug of choice. You should have about 1 ounce of lavender simple syrup.
3. Brew coffee or espresso into the mug containing the simple syrup, and add CBD oil.
4. If you have a milk steamer, steam milk and pour it over the coffee. If you don't have a milk steamer on hand, pour the milk into a blender, add the coffee with lavender and CBD oil, and blend until frothy, then return to the coffee mug. Serve immediately.

Supergood Golden Milk

If you had to make a list of superfoods, turmeric might just be number one. It's full of antioxidants and has been shown to help with illnesses ranging from depression to arthritis to blood clots. Like CBD, studies suggest that it may also have anticancer properties. Golden milk is an ancient Ayurvedic tradition that combines turmeric, black pepper, and warm milk to make a super-soothing tonic. This recipe is by Ashlae Warner, the creator of the popular wellness blog Oh, Ladycakes *and the founder of Supergood hemp products, one of which is a CBD-infused golden milk powder. Genius.*

SERVES 1

Ingredients

1½ cups unsweetened almond milk

1 tablespoon coconut butter

2 teaspoons Supergood golden powder (about 20 mg); you can also use any CBD oil and a golden milk powder

1 to 3 teaspoons maple syrup

Pinch of fine sea salt

Blender Method

1. Add the milk to a small saucepan. Cook on medium heat just until it starts to steam, then turn off the heat and set the milk aside for a few minutes to cool.
2. Place the coconut butter, golden powder, maple syrup, and salt in a blender, then cover with the warm milk.
3. Blend on high speed until smooth and creamy, 1 to 2 minutes, depending on the blender. Enjoy immediately.

continued

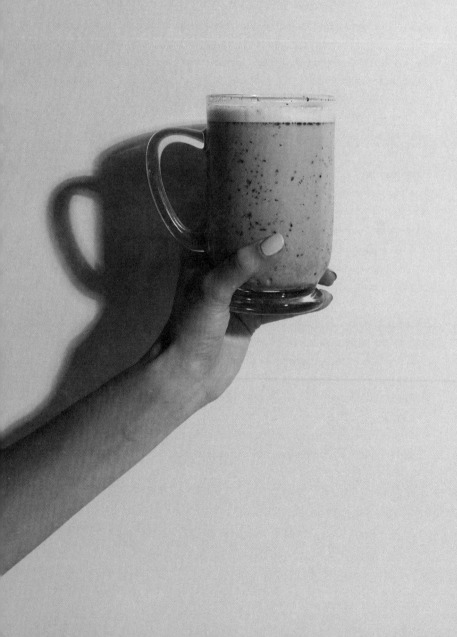

Mug Method

1. Add the milk to a small saucepan. Cook on medium heat just until it starts to steam, then turn off the heat and set the milk aside for a few minutes to cool.
2. Place the coconut butter, golden powder, maple syrup, and sea salt in a 16-ounce mug. Slowly pour the warm milk into the mug and whisk to combine. Enjoy immediately.

If cold Golden Milk is desired, chill in the refrigerator and enjoy within 48 hours.

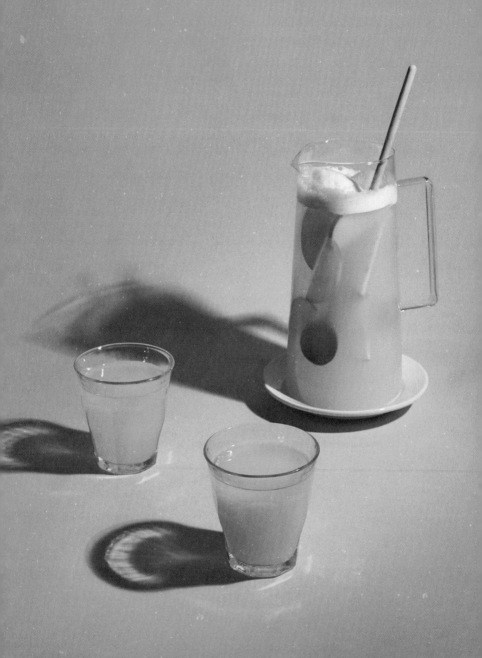

Nausea-Kicking Ginger Tonic

Had a little too much fun at happy hour yesterday? Going on a road trip and worried about getting carsick? This is your new go-to tonic. It's a little bit spicy, very refreshing, and the combination of ginger and sparkling water is guaranteed to calm your stomach. Ginger is famous for its anti-nausea properties and has even been studied as a complementary treatment for people going through chemotherapy, which can cause debilitating nausea. Couple that with the nausea-fighting properties of CBD, and you might actually start to enjoy road trips. You can make this one with just the ginger and apple, or add a little bit of fennel herbal extract for some extra inner-ear-supporting power.

SERVES 2

Ingredients

24 ounces cold sparkling water

1 medium hand of ginger, juiced
   (or about 2 ounces ginger juice)

1 green apple, juiced (or about
   2 ounces apple juice), plus ¼
   apple, thinly sliced, for garnish

2 doses (about 30 mg) CBD oil
   (I like Lord Jones Lemon-
   Flavored Pain & Wellness
   Tincture)

Optional superfood boost: Single
   dose of fennel herbal extract

Method

1. Pour the sparkling water into a large carafe or mason jar.
2. Juice the fresh ginger and apple and add to the carafe.
3. Add the CBD oil and optional fennel extract.
4. Stir with a large spoon until fully incorporated. Add some thinly sliced apples, using about ¼ an apple, for a fun twist.
5. Store in the fridge and drink throughout the day, or pour over ice and bring with you on a road trip.

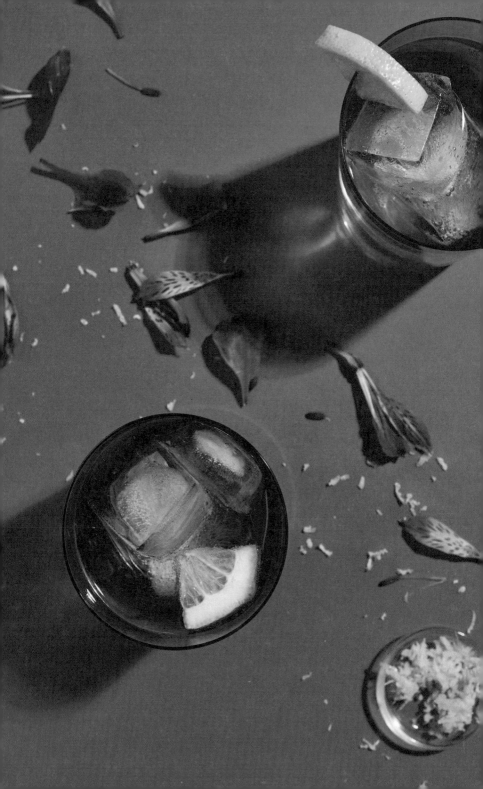

Immune-Boosting Elderberry Shrub

Whenever I'm getting sick, people start offering me bone broth, tea, and soup. But for some reason, all I ever want is something cold! This immune-boosting elderberry shrub is my new favorite "I feel a cold coming on" ritual. Vinegar, especially apple cider vinegar, is thought to boost the immune system; honey is great for soothing the throat; and elderberry is nothing less than a celebrity when it comes to immune-boosting herbs. Elderberry syrup will be on the shelf of most health food stores, but my favorite product is from Gaia Herbs. For an optional immune-supporting superfood boost, add some Echinacea extract. CBD provides that last little bit of immune-supporting plant power, making this the perfect drink to turn to when you feel that first scratch in your throat.

SERVES 3

Syrup Ingredients

5 tablespoons apple cider vinegar

4 tablespoons filtered water

4 teaspoons elderberry syrup

3 teaspoons grated lemon zest

4 doses (about 60 mg) CBD-infused honey (I like Luce Farm hemp honey) *or* 4 doses CBD oil and 3 tablespoons honey

Shrub Ingredients

48 ounces sparkling water (16 ounces for each shrub)

Optional superfood boost: One dose (this will vary depending on the type of herbal extract used, but is usually about 1 mL) of echinacea herbal extract (I like the brand Herb Pharm for these tinctures)

Method

1. Place the vinegar and water in a small saucepan and heat to a simmer.

continued

2. Add elderberry syrup and lemon zest, stirring until totally combined. Let the mixture sit with the lid on and cool for about 5 minutes.

3. Add CBD-infused honey and stir. This makes enough syrup for three shrubs, so either use immediately or store in fridge.

4. To finish the shrub, pour 16 ounces of sparkling water into a glass with ice, and add one-third of the elderberry mixture and the optional superfood boost, if using. Stir completely until it's slightly foamy at the top. Serve immediately.

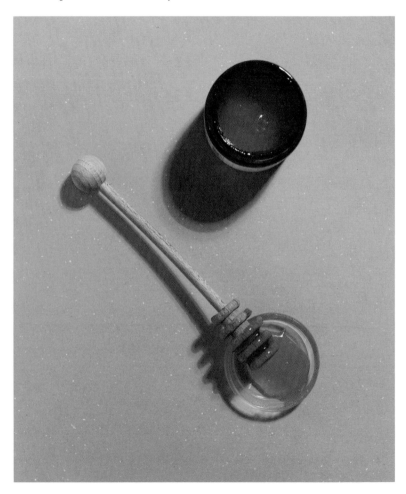

Mint Chip Afternoon Smoothie

Ahhh, the dreaded 3 p.m. slump. It's been hours since lunch and there are still hours to go until dinner. Where do you turn? If you're like most people, you're craving chocolate, a cookie, or a coffee the size of your head. Luckily, you now have this amazing smoothie to turn to. Mint is so invigorating, and cacao nibs are naturally caffeinated to get you through the rest of the day. It tastes a bit like mint chocolate chip ice cream, but it's full of healthy fats and veggies, so there's no reason to feel guilty about having this smoothie any day of the week. For an extra superfood boost, add some grass-fed collagen; it's soothing to the digestive tract and the joints and adds to the thick, creamy texture of this smoothie.

SERVES 1

Ingredients

1 large frozen banana

1 cup fresh spinach

1 cup unsweetened almond milk

½ medium avocado

¼ cup fresh mint leaves (make sure to remove the stems— they're really bitter!)

1 dose (about 15 mg) CBD oil (I like Green Mountain CBD's chocolate mint hemp oil)

½ cup cacao nibs, plus more for garnish (I like Navitas Organics cacao nibs)

Optional superfood boost: One serving (2 scoops) of Vital Proteins unflavored Grass Fed Collagen

Method

1. Add the frozen banana, spinach, almond milk, avocado, mint leaves, and CBD oil to the blender. Blend on low until all the big items are broken down. Then turn to high and blend until there aren't any clumps and the consistency is nice and thick, like soft-serve ice cream.

continued

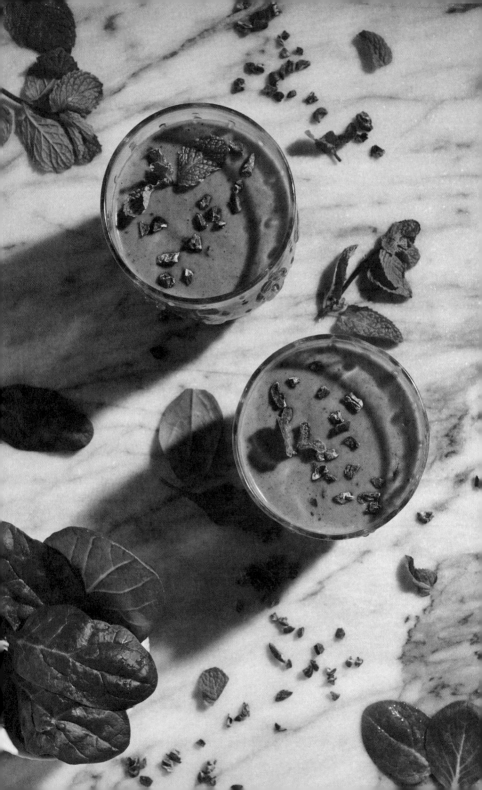

2. Add cacao nibs and pulse until they are dispersed but not blended; you want them there to add texture and crunch!

3. Pour into your smoothie glass and top with a few cacao nibs. Serve immediately. Deliciously thick and creamy, the best way to have this smoothie is with a spoon!

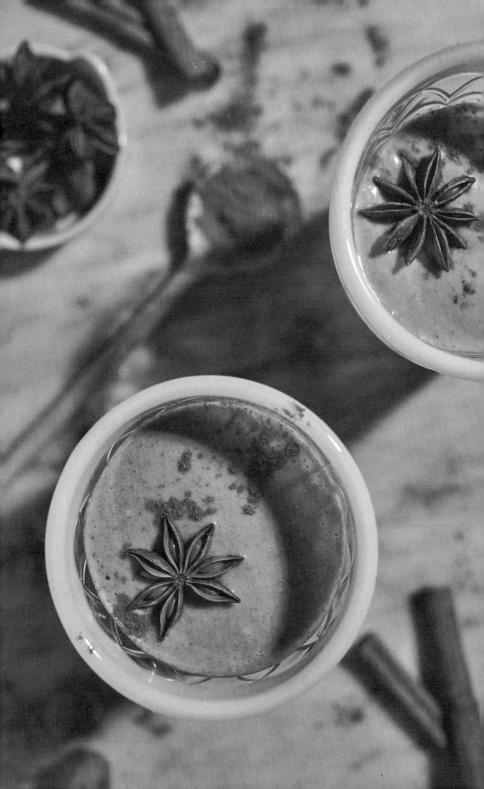

Peanut Butter Chai Morning Smoothie

On the anti-inflammatory food pyramid, there's an entire space dedicated to herbs and spices. This is because many of them have extremely potent anti-inflammatory properties. Unfortunately, if you're constantly on the go and aren't frequently making curries, soups, or other meals that require a bunch of spices, it can be hard to get your recommended daily dose. This slightly unconventional smoothie solves that problem. It contains turmeric, ginger, star anise, nutmeg, cinnamon, and all the spices in chai tea—which are balanced out nicely by a big glob of peanut butter and banana.

SERVES 1

Ingredients

1 cup unsweetened nondairy milk
  (I use coconut milk)

¼ teaspoon turmeric

¼ teaspoon Ceylon cinnamon

⅛ teaspoon nutmeg

⅛ teaspoon ground ginger

1 whole star anise piece

1 chai tea bag (I use a black tea, but you can also use an herbal chai)

1 tablespoon chia seeds

1 large frozen banana

1 heaping tablespoon organic peanut butter

1 dose (about 15 mg) CBD oil (I like to use one that has turmeric in it)

Method

1. Heat the milk in a small saucepan until steam starts rising. Add turmeric, cinnamon, nutmeg, ginger, and star anise, and stir until there are no clumps.
2. Turn off the heat and add the chai tea bag and chia seeds. Cover and allow to cool completely.
3. Remove the tea bag and pour the milk into a blender. Add frozen banana, peanut butter, and CBD oil, and blend on high.
4. Pour into your favorite smoothie glass, top with a few extra chia seeds, and serve immediately.

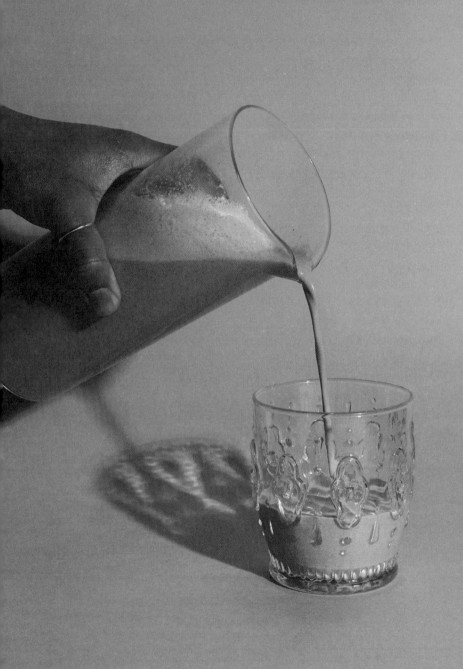

Sedona Magic Mylk

If you know anything about Sedona, Arizona, you know that it's a hot spot for all things health and wellness, self-care, energy healing, crystal healing, aura reading—I think you get the idea. It also happens to be my hometown. Whenever I'm back, I make a daily trip to the Local Juicery for smoothies, juices, acai bowls, treats, and snacks. Recently, they started making a bright blue CBD-infused Magic Mylk. I played with the idea of doing a recipe inspired by this sweet and ever so slightly salty drink, but honestly, it's perfect just the way it is. I love using the CBD brand 2Rise Naturals for this one, since the founder is also from Sedona and it's one of the best-tasting CBDs I've encountered.

SERVES 2

Ingredients

4 cups water

1 cup cashew or hemp seeds

½ teaspoon Blue Majik spirulina

¼ cup maple syrup

1 dropper 2Rise Naturals THC-Free CBD Oil Tincture

½ teaspoon vanilla extract

¼ teaspoon pink Himalayan salt

4 cups coconut water

Method

1. In a high-speed blender, combine water and cashew or hemp seeds, Blue Majik spirulina, maple syrup, CBD, vanilla, and pink salt.
2. Blend on high for 1 to 2 minutes until very creamy. There is no need to strain this milk so long as it is very well blended.

Once it is well combined, pour into a large pitcher or two glasses and add the coconut water. Stir with a large spoon and enjoy!

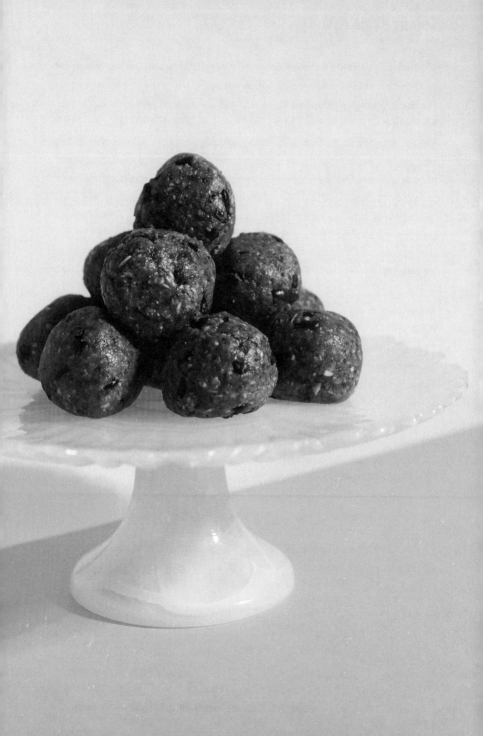

SWEETS, SNACKS, AND COCKTAILS

Cookie Dough Bites

Let's not beat around the bush—granola bars are objectively delicious. I'd eat them for two meals a day if I could. Sadly, they're oftentimes loaded with sugar and a bunch of other ingredients I can't pronounce. This is why homemade energy bites are one of my favorite wellness inventions of all time. These are made to taste like cookie dough (and they actually do) but are nice and low in sugar and high in fiber and healthy fats, making them a great snack to pair with coffee or a CBD Oil London Fog (page 107), just sayin'. They take about 10 minutes to make, so they're the perfect way to get your daily dose of hemp-based wellness. As soon as I perfected this recipe, they became an integral part of my weekly routine, and I hope you'll add them to yours, too.

MAKES ABOUT 10 BITES

Ingredients

½ cup organic, gluten-free oats

½ cup raw walnuts or pecans, unsalted

¼ cup coarsely ground flaxseeds

4 medium-sized dates

2 tablespoons cashew butter

1 tablespoon coconut butter

1 teaspoon vanilla extract

½ teaspoon ground cinnamon

¼ teaspoon salt

10 doses (about 150 mg) CBD oil (I like Mana Artisan Botanics Hawaiian Turmeric Hemp Oil for this recipe because the CBD is in macadamia nut oil)

4 tablespoons cacao nibs

Method

1. Add oats, walnuts or pecans, and flaxseeds to a food processor. Pulse about 10 times for 1 or 2 seconds each.
2. Add the rest of the ingredients except the cacao nibs to the processor and pulse 5 to 10 times until the new ingredients are mixed. Take a

continued

spatula to the sides of the processor to make sure all ingredients are getting hit by the blade, then pulse again, about 5 times this time for 4 or 5 seconds each. You want the consistency to be a chunky paste, not totally smooth.

3. Remove the mixture from the food processor and put in a medium-sized mixing bowl.

4. Fold in the cacao nibs (like you do with chocolate chip cookies) with a spatula until evenly distributed.

5. Divide dough into 10 even sections and roll each into a ball about the size of a Ping-Pong ball.

6. Store in the freezer, and when you're ready to eat, just allow about 10 minutes for them to thaw before enjoying.

Chocolate-Raspberry Mousse

If you ask my dad, he'll tell you that the flavor combination of dark chocolate and raspberry is the most delicious in the world. And I'd have to agree! (He's a wise man.) Lucky for all of us, both cacao powder and berries are chock-full of antioxidants, which means they protect our body from oxidative stress—just like CBD. Therefore, the antioxidant power of this super-decadent dessert is off the charts. This mousse is best made with super-sweet raspberries that are in season. (Berries are one of those foods that you should always try to buy organic, and that's because they have no skin or peel to protect them from pesticides.) If they're on the bland side, try adding some maple syrup and sweeten to taste.

SERVES 2

Ingredients

½ cup cashews, soaked overnight

1 tablespoon chia seeds, soaked overnight

1 whole avocado

About 15 raspberries, plus a few more for garnish

½ cup cacao powder

½ teaspoon vanilla extract

2 doses (about 30 mg) of your favorite CBD oil

1 to 2 tablespoons maple syrup (optional)

1 tablespoon hemp seeds, for garnish

Method

1. Strain water from the cashews and chia seeds and place them in a blender.
2. Add the avocado, raspberries, cacao powder, vanilla, and CBD oil to the blender, and blend until it reaches a creamy, mousse-like texture. You might have to pause and redistribute the ingredients a few times.

continued

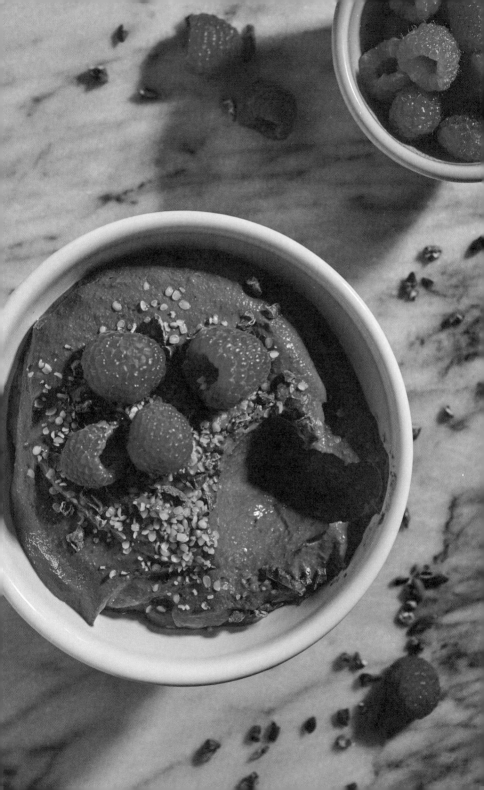

3. Do a quick taste test. If the raspberries you used were nice and sweet, the mousse might be perfect as is. If not, add ½ tablespoon of maple syrup, blend, and taste again. Keep adding ½ teaspoon at a time until you're happy with the level of sweetness.

4. Using a spatula, place mousse into two small glass ramekins. Top with hemp seeds and fresh raspberries. Serve immediately or chill in the fridge and enjoy over the next few days.

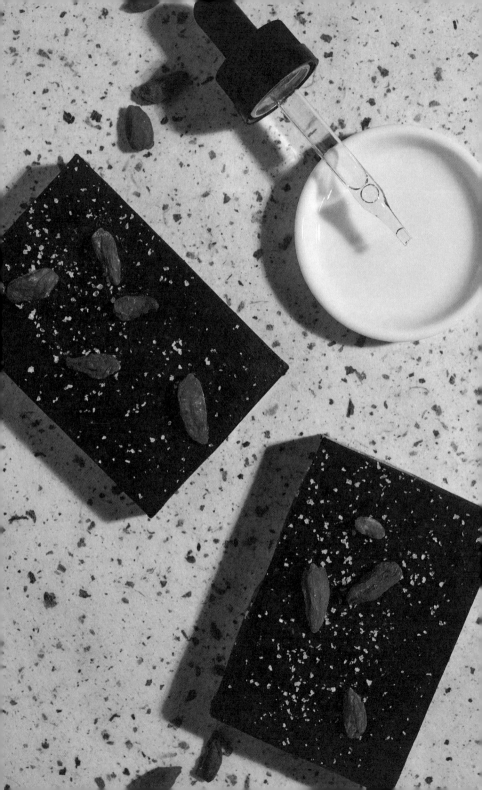

Superfood Chocolate Bars

There's nothing better than a big slice of dark chocolate after lunch or dinner, and these freezer chocolates are no exception. The strong taste of cacao powder easily masks the taste of the reds powder, and the goji berries and coconut add a little texture and crunch. These chocolates are shockingly easy to make, and can be stored in the freezer for whenever a chocolate craving hits. I recommend getting a silicone chocolate bar mold (you can also use a soap mold)—they are super cheap and make the whole process so much easier—but if you don't have one, you can use a small Pyrex dish and then use a knife to cut them into two bars or six smaller pieces of chocolate.

SERVES ABOUT 6

Ingredients

⅓ cup cacao butter

1 tablespoon coconut oil, plus more to brush on

¼ cup cacao powder

3 teaspoons reds powder or acai powder

2 tablespoons dried goji berries (no added sugar)

1 tablespoon unsweetened shredded coconut

6 doses (about 90 mg) CBD oil

Coarse sea salt, for garnish

Method

1. Melt the cacao butter and coconut oil in a double boiler until there are no clumps.
2. Slowly pour in the cacao powder and reds powder and whisk until fully incorporated.
3. Remove from heat and fold in goji berries, coconut, and CBD oil.
4. Pour the mixture into silicone chocolate bar molds.
5. Allow bars to cool in the freezer until hardened.
6. Remove bars from freezer, brush lightly with coconut oil, and sprinkle with salt.
7. Return bars to the freezer (about an hour) and serve them whenever a chocolate craving hits. Just allow 5 to 10 minutes for them to soften.

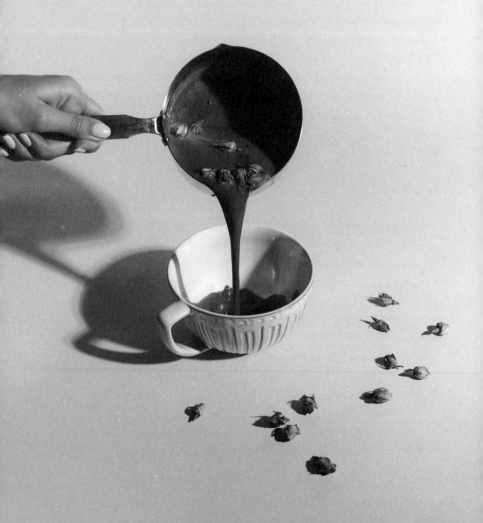

Adaptogenic Hot Chocolate

This recipe was developed by my friends and fellow CBD experts at The Alchemist's Kitchen, a store and café in NYC that really knows how to celebrate the healing power of plants. The herbalists who work there are crazy about CBD, and even better, they're crazy about educating people about CBD. With adaptogenic herbs to nourish the nervous system and balance cortisol levels—and CBD to relieve inflammation, pain, stress, and anxiety—this rich and delicious beverage will help you to breeze through your day feeling balanced and relaxed. Plus, who doesn't love hot chocolate? I've been replacing my afternoon coffee with this awesome recipe.

SERVES 1

Ingredients

1 cup full-fat coconut milk

2 teaspoons cacao powder

1 teaspoon ashwagandha powder

1 teaspoon turmeric

½ teaspoon powdered cardamom

½ teaspoon cinnamon, plus more
    for garnish

½ teaspoon vanilla extract

15 drops of 500 mg Plant Alchemy
    CBD oil (30 mg in total)

1 tablespoon rose petals or buds
    for garnish

Method

1. Heat the coconut milk in a small saucepan.
2. In your mug, combine cacao, ashwagandha, turmeric, cardamom, and cinnamon.
3. Pour the heated coconut milk over the powders in your mug while gently whisking the beverage.
4. Add the vanilla and CBD oil, and whisk further to fully blend all ingredients.
5. Top beverage with rose buds and a shake of cinnamon. Enjoy!

Recipe by Emily Berg, resident herbalist at The Alchemist's Kitchen, New York

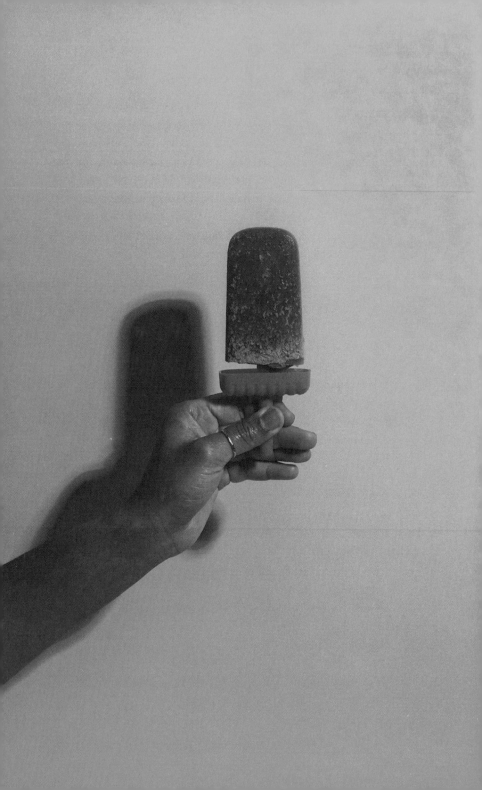

Bulletproof Latte Pops

My friend Liz is the healthy-Popsicle queen. She authored the cookbook Glow Pops *as well as the upcoming cookbook* Healthier Together, *and she is an endless supply of insanely delicious recipes and knowledge about health and nutrition. She also just so happens to be obsessed with CBD oil. The best part about Popsicles is that you can store them in the fridge and eat them at any time. These are perfect when you want a cold, invigorating treat without all the sugar. I plan to keep them in my freezer all summer long.*

MAKES 5 TO 6 POPS

Ingredients

¾ cup full-fat coconut milk

¾ cup bottled cold brew coffee concentrate (do not dilute with water as the bottle instructs)

¼ cup coconut syrup (can substitute maple syrup or honey)

2 tablespoons MCT oil

6 doses (about 90 mg) neutral-flavored CBD oil

½ teaspoon ground cinnamon (optional, but adds a lovely kick)

Method

1. Put all the ingredients in a blender and blend until very smooth; you can also do this in a mixing bowl with a spatula or whisk.
2. Pour the mixture into molds and freeze for 1 hour, then insert sticks and freeze for at least 4 more hours, or until solid.

You can also make these pops caffeine-free by boiling 1 cup of water, then adding 3 rooibos tea bags (or 3 teaspoons of loose-leaf rooibos) and covering. Let steep for 10 minutes, then discard the bags (or strain the tea, if using loose leaf). Measure out ¾ cup of tea and substitute it for cold brew concentrate.

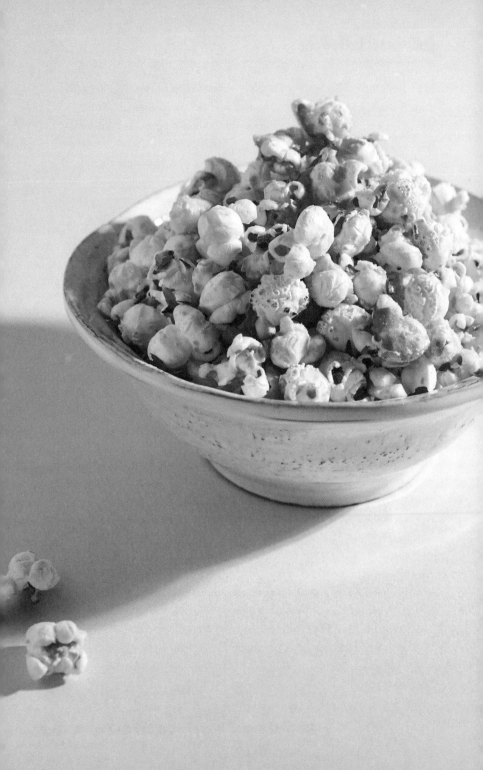

Chile Cheese Popcorn

Is there anything better than sitting down on a Sunday afternoon with a giant bowl of popcorn and a movie you've been dying to see? It's one of my favorite rituals. Sadly, most of the popcorns out there are less than healthy and leave you feeling like a big bowl of butter for the rest of the day. That's why I designed this popcorn recipe with homemade CBD chile oil, plus nutritional yeast for some extra cheesy goodness. Nutritional yeast has a natural cheesy flavor, but it's dairy-free, high in protein and fiber, and full of B vitamins.

SERVES 1

Chile Oil Ingredients

2 tablespoons olive oil

1 tablespoon chile flakes

1 dose (about 15 mg) neutral-flavored CBD oil

Popcorn Ingredients

1 tablespoon coconut oil

½ cup unpopped non-GMO popcorn kernels

2 tablespoons nutritional yeast

1 teaspoon sea salt

Method

1. Combine olive oil, chile flakes, and CBD oil in a small container and allow to sit for at least 3 hours or up to overnight.
2. Melt coconut oil on medium heat in a large saucepan.
3. Add 3 or 4 popcorn kernels and cover the pan with a lid, shaking it so the kernels slide back and forth in the bottom of the pan.
4. Wait for the kernels to pop, and then add in the rest of the kernels. Keep shaking the pan with the lid closed and wait until the whole pan fills up with popped kernels.
5. Pour popcorn into your biggest bowl and quickly (while popcorn is still hot) drizzle chile oil and nutritional yeast on top. If you really enjoy spicy popcorn, you can pour extra chile flakes in, too.
6. Use your hands to toss the popcorn to distribute the spices evenly. Add salt to taste.

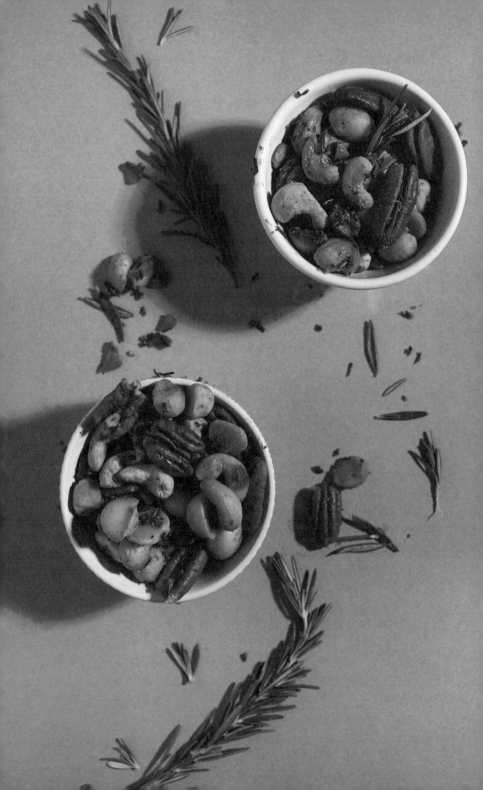

Rosemary Toasted Nuts

A few years ago, results from a study conducted in the UK showed that rosemary was able to help improve memory. Quickly, rosemary products started flying off the shelves until most health food stores were completely sold out. To this day, if I'm working on something that requires a lot of brainpower (like writing a book, for example), I diffuse rosemary essential oil in my apartment. But by combining CBD oil and rosemary, you're making the perfect snack to fuel your brain. You won't hate how your kitchen smells, either.

MAKES 1½ CUPS TOASTED NUTS

Ingredients

1½ cups raw unsalted nuts of your choice (I use macadamia nuts, pecans, and cashews)

1 tablespoon ghee

2 teaspoons fresh chopped rosemary leaves

1 dose (about 15 mg) CBD oil (I like Charlotte's Web Hemp Extract Oil in olive oil)

Fine sea salt

Method

1. Preheat oven to 325°F and spread nuts in an even layer on a baking sheet.
2. Bake for about 10 minutes, until some of the nuts are golden and a nice toasted aroma is coming out of the oven. You're going to put the nuts on heat later, so better to underroast them than overroast them at this point.
3. Heat the ghee and rosemary in a skillet over medium heat, stirring occasionally until you start smelling rosemary wafting from the pan.
4. Add the nuts and stir until the ghee completely coats them. Leave them in the skillet, stirring regularly, for a few more minutes, until the nuts are golden brown, and add the CBD oil. Then pour onto a paper towel–topped baking pan. Add sea salt to taste.
5. Allow to cool about 10 minutes and then snack away.

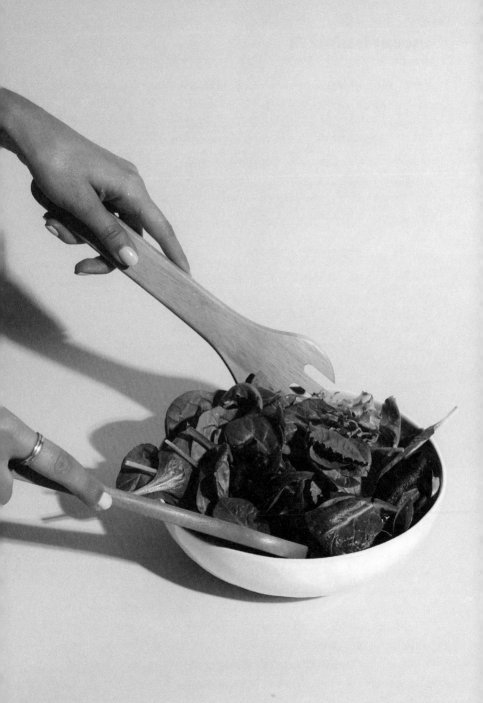

Avocado Dill Dressing

It's so easy to default to buying premade salad dressings, even though they're typically full of sugar and preservatives and unhealthy fats. I was guilty of this for years; that is, until I realized how much more delicious it is to make dressings yourself. The fact that they are healthier and cheaper is just an added bonus. This dressing goes with any type of lettuce and features healthy fats and fresh herbs. Lemon is the obvious choice, but lime is just as delicious.

SERVES 1

Ingredients

½ ripe avocado

½ medium lime, juiced

1 tablespoon olive oil

½ teaspoon dried dill

Pinch of salt

Pinch of pepper

1 dose (about 15 mg) CBD oil in olive oil base

Method

1. Slice the avocado in half, and using a spoon, remove the inside from the half without the pit. Place it in the bottom of an empty salad bowl. (Store the other half in the fridge with the pit still in it; this will help keep it fresh.)
2. Add lime juice, olive oil, dill, salt, pepper, and CBD oil to the bowl.
3. Using a fork, mash the avocado into the bottom of the bowl, mixing it thoroughly with the other ingredients.
4. You can mash until the dressing is totally smooth, or you can leave some nice chunks of avocado. Then add whatever greens you're using, and toss them in the dressing right in the salad bowl.

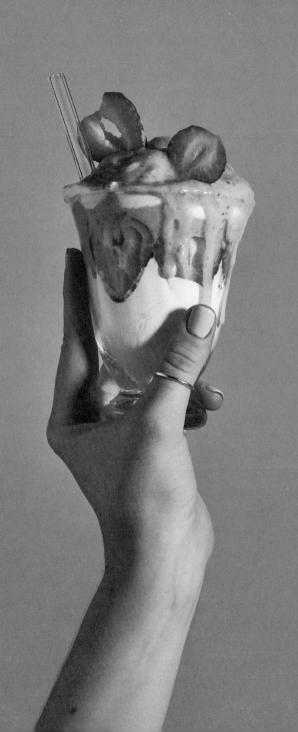

Vegan Strawberry Milkshake

As someone who's very sensitive to dairy, I've been left out of milkshakes pretty much all my life. They are basically a dairy bomb, after all. But this recipe is made from dairy-free ice cream, coconut milk whipped cream, and frozen strawberries. It's delicious, decadent, and most importantly, completely free of dairy. It also features hemp seeds, which are high in essential fatty acids and minerals like potassium, magnesium, and zinc. I like having this one in an old-fashioned milkshake glass.

SERVES 1

Milkshake Ingredients

½ cup hemp seeds, soaked
overnight in about 1 cup water

2 cups frozen strawberries

½ cup dairy-free vanilla ice cream

1 dose (about 15 mg) CBD oil

Whipped Cream Ingredients

2¾ ounces organic heavy coconut
cream

1 teaspoon coconut sugar

½ teaspoon vanilla extract

Method

1. Add the hemp seeds and soaking water to the blender and blend until you get a creamy, milk-like consistency.
2. Add frozen strawberries and ice cream. Blend again. Add the CBD oil. This should be nice and thick from the frozen fruit. Transfer to a mixing bowl using a spatula.
3. Pour the coconut cream into the blender and add coconut sugar and vanilla extract. Blend until fluffy and creamy. Transfer to a mixing bowl.
4. In a medium glass, pour a layer of coconut cream in the bottom, top with a layer of strawberry milkshake, and repeat until the glass is overflowing with creamy strawberry deliciousness. Serve immediately.

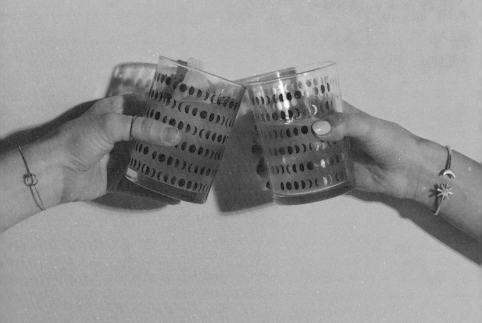

CBD-Infused After-Dinner Drink

Bitter herbs are one of my favorite wellness secrets. I use them before almost every meal to stimulate digestion, and if I've eaten a little too much or something that doesn't agree with me, I'll follow my meal with bitters as well. Cut to this healthy after-dinner cocktail, perfect for those three-hour-long dinner parties when no one is quite ready to go home yet. I use my favorite bourbon or whiskey, an orange squeeze for a little sweetness, and a dropperful of Cordial Organics Celebrate Bitters, which already have CBD in them. If you don't want to use this specific product, go ahead and use some regular aromatic bitters and your favorite CBD oil.

SERVES 2

Ingredients

2 ounces bourbon or rye

2 dropperfuls Cordial Organics
    Celebrate Bitters (or a few shakes of
    aromatic bitters and 1 dose of your
    favorite neutral-flavored CBD oil)

½ medium orange, cut into two slices

Method

1. Fill two glasses with ice and pour 1 ounce of bourbon or rye into each.
2. Add a few drops of bitters, and squeeze juice from an orange quarter into each glass.
3. Stir and serve immediately.

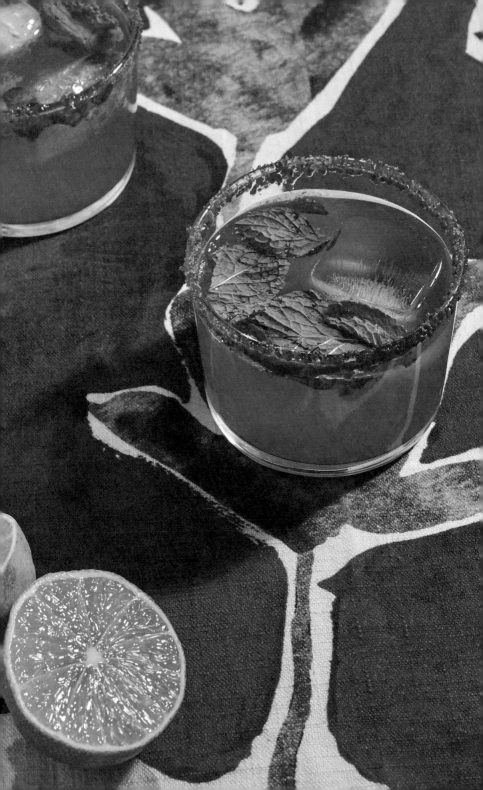

Prickly Pear Mojito

There's nothing better than a fun, fruity, wonderfully pink cocktail. And luckily, prickly pear also has some cool properties. Research has shown that these fruits can actually help prevent hangovers; Native Americans have long used the fruit and juice as a hangover remedy. When we add the protective powers of CBD to that mix, you might just want to have two or three. If you can't find fresh prickly pear, you can order prickly pear nectar or juice online—just make sure to check out the ingredients and look for one without any added sugar. These fruits are delicious and have enough sweetening power all on their own, especially if you decide to opt for the sugar rim.

SERVES 2

Ingredients

2 teaspoons coconut sugar, plus 3 tablespoons for sugared rim (optional)

1 lime, juiced

10 fresh mint leaves

2 prickly pear fruits or 4 tablespoons prickly pear nectar (I like Arizona Cactus Ranch Prickly Pear Nectar)

2 doses (about 30 mg) of your favorite CBD oil (I like Wildflower CBD + Wellness Tincture in the Tropical Fruit Flavor)

3 ounces white rum of your choice

10 ounces sparkling water

Method

1. For the optional sugared rim, dampen the rims of two cocktail glasses and dip them in 3 tablespoons of coconut sugar.
2. Place the remaining 2 tablespoons of sugar, lime, and mint leaves in the glasses. Using a firm pressing and twisting motion, muddle them together. You can use a designated muddler or just the end of a wooden spoon.

continued

3. Divide the prickly pear nectar and CBD oil between the two glasses.
4. Add 1½ ounces of white rum to each glass, and fill the rest up with sparkling water.
5. Stir thoroughly and enjoy!

If using fresh prickly pear fruits: Store-bought prickly pears are normally already spine-free and can be picked up with your bare hands without a problem, but just to be sure, place the pears in a colander under cold water and swirl them around to get rid of any fine blond hairs that might be lingering. Slice off the thicker skin at both ends of the prickly pear and then remove the rest of the skin (you want to get all the skin off but not so much that you penetrate the seedy area of the fruit). Remove the seeds and blend the fruit in a blender, then add it to the glasses right after you muddle the mint leaves, lime, and sugar.

Gut-Healing Cherry Cardamom Gummies

When you think about edibles, gummies are probably what first pop into your mind. Sadly, visiting a dispensary will reveal some unsightly characters—like high-fructose corn syrup and hydrogenated oils—on the ingredient lists of popular gummies. This recipe is next-level healthy, with grass-fed gelatin (which is great for your gut), real cherries, and fresh spices for a whole food version of your favorite childhood treat. You can put these in cute gummy molds or simply pour them into a Pyrex dish and slice into evenly sized squares.

SERVES 5

Ingredients

1 bag (16 ounces) frozen organic cherries

½ teaspoon almond extract

¼ teaspoon cardamom

⅛ teaspoon salt

¼ cup grass-fed gelatin (I recommend Vital Proteins Beef Gelatin)

5 doses (about 75 mg) neutral-flavored CBD oil

Method

1. Heat the cherries, almond extract, cardamom, and salt over medium heat in a medium saucepan, mushing the cherries as you go.
2. Cook until mixture is mostly liquid, with just a few chunks of cherry left, 5 or 10 minutes.
3. Turn off the heat and let the mixture cool slightly, then transfer it to a blender and blend on high until it looks like juice.
4. Return the mixture to the saucepan and check to make sure it's warm to the touch but not boiling. If it's cooled off too much, you can just reheat it for a few minutes.
5. Turn on the heat to medium and slowly, a little bit at a time, add the gelatin, whisking constantly. With the last bit of gelatin, add the

continued

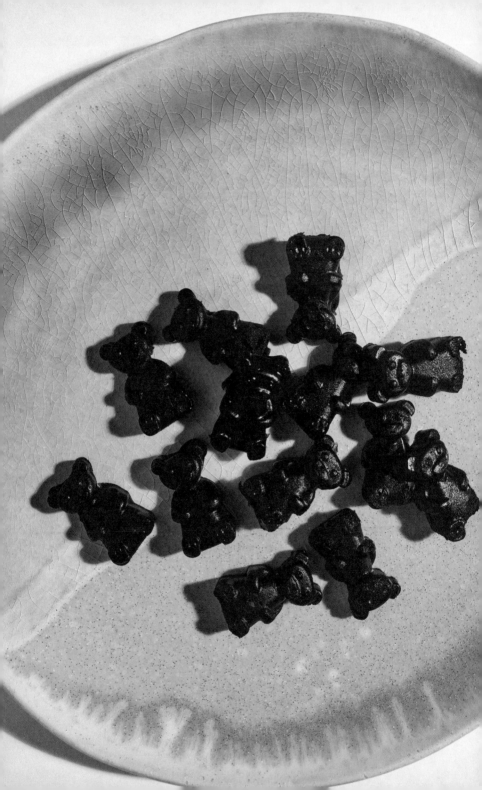

CBD oil and whisk thoroughly, making sure there are no clumps of gelatin sticking to the bottom of the pan. Turn off the heat.

6. You can pour the entire mixture into a Pyrex dish to cut into squares later, or you can use a dropper and silicone gummy mold of your choice—just pay attention to dosing and make sure you separate your final gummies into 5 different servings.

7. If you're using a gummy mold and dropper, make sure you tap the dropper on the side of the pan every time you transfer to reduce spillage. The transferring will get more difficult as the gelatin mixture cools off, so keep up the pace if you can.

8. Make sure each individual gummy mold is completely filled up, then pop in the fridge and let them set, about 2 hours. You can store gummies in the fridge for 3 to 4 days.

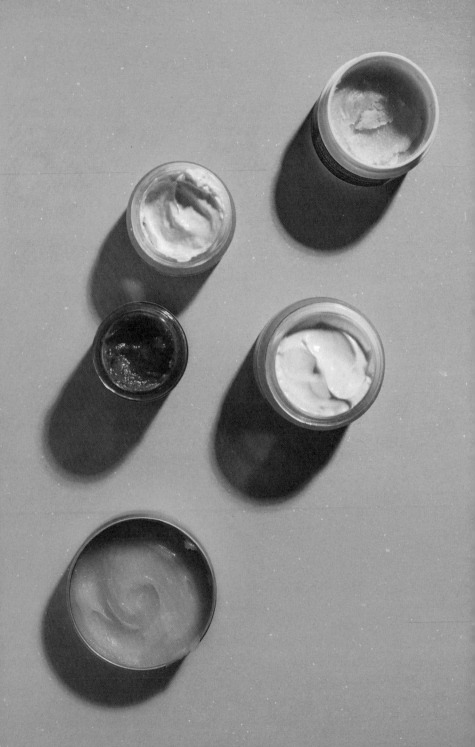

CBD Self-Care: Ten Ways to Bring CBD Into Your Routine

As delightful as it is to infuse popcorn, coffee, and gummies with CBD, it's even more fun to incorporate it into your self-care routine. Luckily, many companies are starting to make CBD-based balms, body oils, face oils, lotions, and creams—all of which can be used in these recipes. So feel free to mix and match, and don't stress too much about what form of topical CBD product I've recommended in the recipe; many of them are interchangeable.

As we know, cannabidiol is a potent antioxidant, which means it can be your skin's new best friend. Its apparent anti-inflammatory, anti-itch, and pain-relieving properties also make it the perfect natural remedy for the many topical health woes we all experience. The CBD-inspired rituals that follow may relieve period cramps, give your skin a major antioxidant boost, and turn your bath into a relaxing experience. They may help you alleviate bug bites with bananas, reduce pimples overnight, and soothe a sunburn with 100 percent natural ingredients.

A few of the remedies in this section require glass tincture bottles with a dropper or spray top; you can buy these at most health food stores or anywhere that sells essential oils. Always look for colored glass, as CBD is light sensitive, and store the bottles in a cool, dark place. You'll also need some essential oils and a carrier oil, which is just a neutral-smelling oil used to dilute the strong-smelling essential oils. Most oils will work for this (even coconut oil), but I prefer apricot oil, grape-seed oil, or jojoba oil, as they are liquid at room temperature and relatively inexpensive. I've provided basic dosing information, but remember that dosing CBD—especially in this section, where we're using topical remedies—is more of an art than a science. Other than that, this section is refreshingly straightforward.

Some of the recipes on the following pages are neat, and others involve globbing a bunch of messy ingredients into a big bowl and applying them with your hands. What they all have in common, subject to medical advice, is that they can help you cut down on over-the-counter medications and beauty products with long lists of chemical ingredients. These rituals are simple, wholesome, and will get you in touch with CBD and plant medicine as a whole. Are you ready? Let the relaxation begin!

Overnight Immune Booster

Whether it is vitamin C, bone broth, or an Immune-Boosting Elderberry Shrub (see page 117), everyone seems to have their own go-to remedy for when they start feeling sick. Well, as a health editor, I have an arsenal of them. Applying essential oils to my feet before bed is one of my favorites. Oregano is the perfect choice because of its strong antimicrobial properties, and eucalyptus has been used for centuries as an expectorant (think Vicks VapoRub) and is very soothing to the sinuses and lungs. So give yourself a nice foot rub before bed, don some warm, fuzzy socks, and allow these badass plants to take the reins while you get a good night's sleep.

MAKES 5 TREATMENTS

Ingredients

10 dropperfuls oil of oregano herbal extract (typically, one dropperful is 1 mL or 20 to 30 drops of oregano oil)

5 drops eucalyptus essential oil

5 doses (about 75 mg) CBD oil

1 ounce carrier oil of your choice

Method

1. Add oregano oil to a 1-ounce colored glass spray bottle and follow with eucalyptus oil and CBD oil. Fill the rest of the bottle up with carrier oil.

2. Use this immune booster when you feel those sniffles coming on. Make sure you shake it before you spray, and apply it to your feet (top and bottom). You can also apply this oil to other parts of your body; just steer clear of the face and eyes.

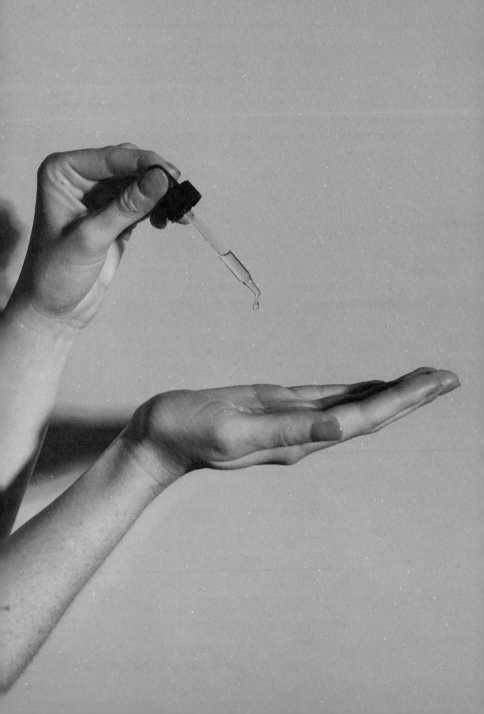

Soothing Sage Belly Rub

Clary sage is one of the most famous essential oils for hormone balance and women's health. It can be a bit strong, in my opinion, so adding lavender essential oil helps tone down the smell and creates a calming blend that feels just medicinal enough. Keep this remedy in a 1-ounce bottle (remember to use colored glass and store in a cool, dry place), and rub generously on your lower belly and lower back during that time of the month. Expert tip: This is best applied after you've just used a warm heating pad on the area or taken an Epsom salt bath.

MAKES 5 TREATMENTS

Ingredients

10 drops clary sage essential oil

2 drops lavender essential oil
   (I like Saje Natural Wellness
   100 percent High Grade
   Lavender Essential Oil)

5 doses (about 75 mg) neutral-
   flavored CBD oil

1 ounce carrier oil of your choice

Method

1. Add clary sage, lavender oil, and CBD oil to a 1-ounce dark-colored glass tincture bottle. Fill to the top with carrier oil.
2. To use, shake the bottle and then cover the palm of your hand in oil, and rub it on your lower abdomen and lower back. Repeat as needed.

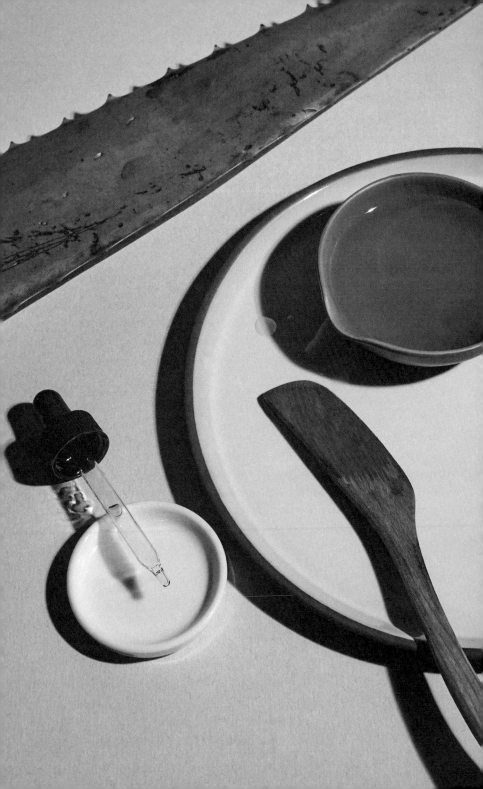

Aloe + CBD Sunburn Gel

No matter how much I stick to the shade, wear protective clothing, and SPF it up when I'm directly in the sun's rays, I occasionally come home a little red. This sunburn gel is my new best friend. With its cooling, calming properties, aloe is a superstar for sunburns, and CBD will work on inflammation, pain, and itching. The peppermint adds a little extra cooling power and makes this remedy smell amazing. A word of caution here: Peppermint is very strong, so don't use more than a few drops. If you're planning to put this on your face or anywhere near your eyes, use half the peppermint oil, because it can irritate your eyes, and make sure to wash your hands after you apply it.

MAKES 1 TREATMENT

Ingredients

¼ cup aloe vera gel (you can buy this at a health food store)

1 dose (about 15 mg) CBD oil, preferably in coconut oil

3 to 5 drops peppermint essential oil

Method

1. Mix aloe gel with CBD oil in a small mixing bowl.
2. Add peppermint oil and mix thoroughly.
3. Apply gently to the affected area.

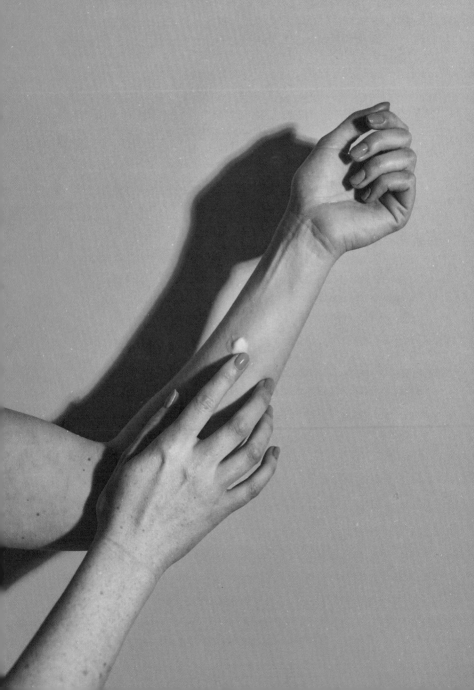

Banana Peel Bug Bite Remedy

Bug bites are the worst. They're red and itchy, and they seem to flare up as soon as you lay your head down to go to sleep. Banana peels have been used in folk medicine for years to treat bug bites; baking soda and witch hazel are great for itchiness; and as we already know, CBD works on itches, inflammation, and pain. This remedy will take the form of a thick white paste and will harden right on your skin in 5 to 10 minutes. Feel free to leave it on there as long as you want; this will help keep you from scratching, which I know is hard to resist, even though you know it only makes things worse.

TREATS 5 BUG BITES (or if you're like me, just one that has swollen to the size of a silver dollar)

Ingredients

1 banana peel

2 teaspoons baking soda

1 dose (about 15 mg) neutral-flavored CBD oil

2½ teaspoons witch hazel

Method

1. Use a butter knife to scrape off 1 teaspoon of the white pulp on the inside of the banana peel, and transfer it to a small mixing bowl. Add baking soda, CBD oil, and witch hazel, and whisk until the mixture forms a thick paste. If it's too dry, just add a little more witch hazel. If it looks a little too liquidy, that's okay. It will be harder than you think and stay put once it's on your skin.

2. Smear a thick layer onto your nastiest bug bite right away and let it dry.

3. When you're ready to remove the paste, just wipe off with a warm, wet washcloth.

4. You can store extra paste in an airtight container for a few hours to apply again, but this one is best made fresh each day.

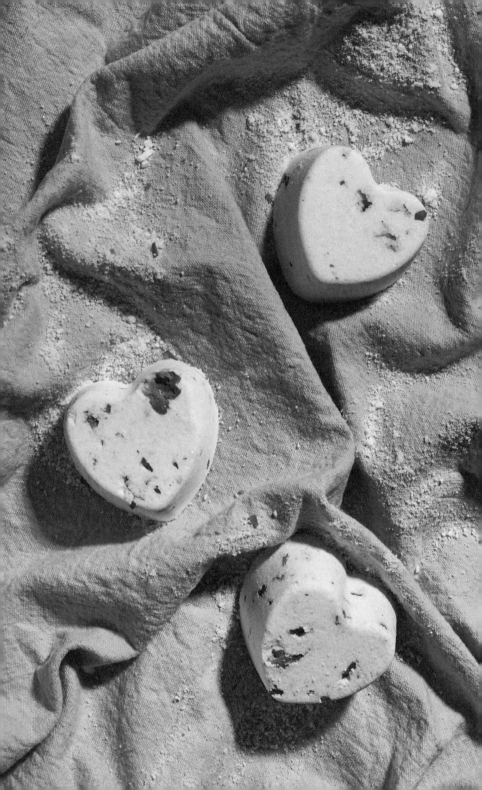

Coconut Rose Bath Bomb

If you're lucky enough to have a bathtub, a bath bomb is the perfect way to give your skin a nice dose of cannabidiol. They're surprisingly easy to make and a fun way to turn a normal bath into a healing ritual. This recipe combines the romantic smell of rose with the soothing properties of coconut oil. Rose has a nice, subtle scent, so use a neutral CBD oil for this one.

MAKES 4 MEDIUM BATH BOMBS

Ingredients

1 cup baking soda

½ cup citric acid

½ cup Epsom salts

½ cup cornstarch

1 tablespoon coconut oil, melted

4 doses (about 60 mg) CBD oil

1 teaspoon filtered water (don't use more than this)

10 drops rose essential oil

1 small handful of dried rose petals

Method

1. Place baking soda, citric acid, Epsom salts, and cornstarch in a large bowl and mix until well combined.

2. In a small bowl, combine coconut oil, CBD oil, water, and rose essential oil.

3. Slowly pour the wet ingredients into the big bowl with the dry ingredients, and mix thoroughly and evenly with your hands. This part is sometimes easier if you're wearing gloves. The mixture should resemble crumbly sand and should not feel wet to the touch. Once you reach this texture, add the rose petals.

4. Press the mixture firmly into greased molds (you can use bath bomb molds or any muffin pan) and let sit 24 to 48 hours.

5. Once fully dry and hardened, carefully remove bath bombs from the mold.

6. To use a bath bomb, just drop it directly into your bathtub while it's filling up. Store in an airtight container.

Very, Very Green Face Mask

Everyone knows it's healthy to put green things in our bodies through the food we eat, but what about our faces and complexions? Well, you'll be happy to know that skin can benefit from the nutrients in avocado, cucumber, and a little bit of matcha powder as well. That being said, other than CBD, the true superstar ingredient in this mask is Manuka honey, which has been shown to speed wound healing and has even been used in hospitals for that purpose. Many integrative dermatologists recommend Manuka honey masks for acne and other skin issues. This recipe makes enough for two masks, so either do this with a friend or partner (who wants to smear green sludge all over their face alone, anyway?) or keep it in the fridge for a few days.

MAKES 2 MASKS

Ingredients

1 small cucumber with skin on, refrigerated

½ avocado, refrigerated

1 tablespoon Manuka honey

1 teaspoon matcha powder

1 dose (about 15 mg) neutral-flavored CBD oil

Method

1. Slice the cucumber in half and place in a blender. Remove the inside of the avocado and add to the blender.
2. Add honey, matcha powder, and CBD oil to the blender.
3. Blend on low for about a minute. Turn off the blender and use a spatula to wipe down the sides, then run again, this time on high, making sure there aren't any big chunks of cucumber.
4. To use the mask, apply it to your face with a brush, spatula, or your hands. Leave it on for about 10 minutes, and then remove using warm water and a washcloth. Manuka honey is also very hydrating, so you might find that there's no need to moisturize afterward.

Skin-Brightening Probiotic Face Mask

Despite its appearance, this is not the most delicious yogurt parfait you've ever seen. (Although you could definitely eat it if you wanted to!) More and more, research is showing that our skin's microbiome is crucial to overall skin health, and holistic skin-care experts posit that the harsh chemicals in cosmetics and makeup are harming the delicate balance of these bacteria—leading to acne and inflammatory skin conditions like psoriasis. By using kefir—which is a great source of probiotics—you'll be replenishing your skin with good bugs. The addition of mango's exfoliating properties, as well as oats, which are super-calming to the skin, makes this a great mask to use when your skin feels a little dull. This mask looks and tastes and smells a lot like food. And that's what it is—food for your skin.

MAKES 1 MASK

Ingredients

¼ mango

2 tablespoons quick-cook oats

1 tablespoon organic kefir

¼ teaspoon ground ginger

1 dose (about 15 mg) neutral-flavored CBD oil

Method

1. Mash the mango with a fork in the bottom of a small mixing bowl.
2. Add oats, kefir, ginger, and CBD oil, and stir until all the ingredients are distributed evenly.
3. To use the mask, apply it to your face and leave it for about 10 minutes. Be prepared, this one is messy! Remove the mask with warm water.

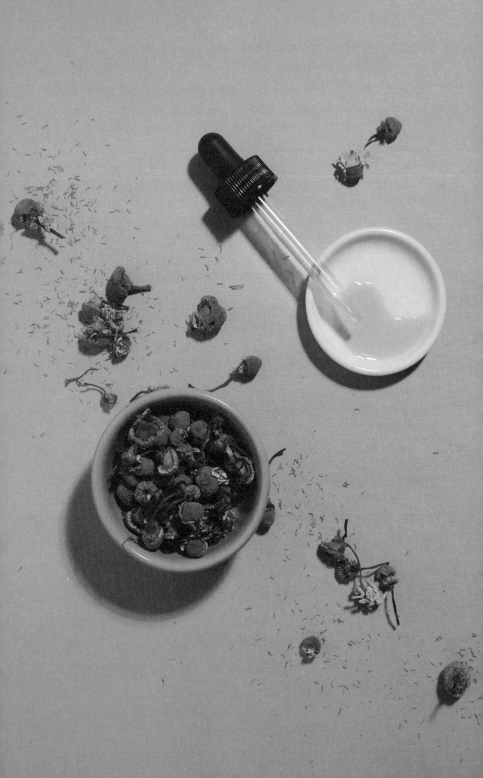

Chamomile-Magnesium Body Oil

Magnesium is often referred to as the relaxation mineral. It plays a role in hundreds of enzymatic reactions in your body that govern everything from your nervous system to the health of your bones. Unfortunately, chronic stress depletes the body's magnesium levels, so a lot of people end up deficient in this important mineral. Luckily, magnesium can be absorbed through the skin, so creating a magnesium body oil with added CBD is a great way to put your feet up and wind down at the end of a long day. A little chamomile extract really brings this oil to the next level, turning it into the perfect ritual to smooth out the tension from the day. An ounce of this oil will contain about 15 mg of CBD and 100 mg of magnesium.

MAKES ABOUT 4 TREATMENTS

Ingredients

400 mg magnesium in a topical magnesium oil spray (I like Life-Flo Pure Magnesium Oil)

4 dropperfuls (about 2,400 mg) chamomile liquid extract

4 doses (about 60 mg) of your favorite CBD oil

2 ounces carrier oil of your choice

Method

1. Combine the magnesium oil, chamomile extract, and CBD oil in a 4-ounce colored glass spray bottle. Fill to the top with carrier oil.
2. To use body oil, shake bottle thoroughly first, and massage oil onto your feet, legs, arms, and the back of your neck before bed. You might notice that this leaves a little bit of white residue on your skin—this is just excess salt and can be easily wiped off in the shower or with a washcloth.

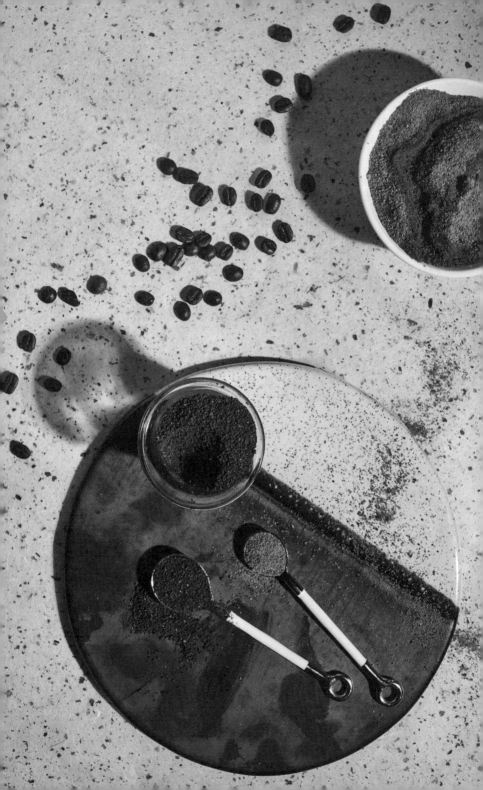

Coffee + CBD Body Scrub

This body scrub is the perfect way to start your morning; it's invigorating, full of antioxidants—from the coffee and the CBD—and leaves your skin smooth as a baby's bottom. It's also ridiculously simple to make; you can even use leftover coffee grounds from your morning cup of joe. I recommend applying this in circular motions all over your body, starting at your feet and working up to your arms and neck (don't forget the backs of your hands!). It's best to do it in the shower right before you wash your body so you minimize the mess and can wash off any stray coffee grounds.

MAKES 1 FULL-BODY SCRUB

Ingredients

¼ cup brown coconut sugar

4 tablespoons coconut oil, melted

1 tablespoon of your favorite ground coffee

2 drops vanilla essential oil

1 dose (about 15 mg) CBD-rich hemp extract

Method

1. Before a shower, combine all ingredients in a mixing bowl until fully incorporated.

2. Apply the scrub to your skin in the shower, scrubbing in a circular motion from your feet all the way up to your neck—and make sure to get the backs of your hands—for silky-smooth skin that smells faintly like an iced latte.

2-Step Spot Treatment

There's nothing worse than using a spot treatment on a pimple only to discover that you've dried out your skin and it's flaking and peeling the next day. Even worse, this excessive dryness will likely trigger more pimples to develop in the same spot. Tea tree oil is an awesome antibacterial, but it and bentonite clay can leave your skin parched. That's why I suggest putting this mask on a pimple first, removing it after 10 or 15 minutes, and then following it up with a CBD balm and vitamin E. The balm is there to help hydrate your skin and fight inflammation while you sleep, and vitamin E is great for scar treatment and prevention.

TREATS 2 TO 3 PIMPLES

Mask Ingredients

¼ teaspoon bentonite clay

¼ teaspoon apple cider vinegar with the "mother" intact (I like Bragg Organic Raw Apple Cider Vinegar)

Balm Ingredients

1 half-pea-size dollop CBD-rich balm (I like Plus CBD Oil Extra-Strength Balm)

1 half-pea-size dollop vitamin E oil

1 drop tea tree essential oil

Method:

1. In a small bowl, combine the bentonite clay and apple cider vinegar. Stir into a thick paste.
2. Apply the mask to your pimple and leave until it is fully dry, 10 to 15 minutes.
3. Remove the mask with warm water and a washcloth.
4. On the back of your hand, mix together the CBD oil balm, vitamin E oil, and tea tree oil until fully blended.
5. Apply the balm directly to your pimple and leave overnight.

A FINAL WORD ON CBD

So there you have it, you're now better equipped to start incorporating CBD into your self-care routine and diet. We've discussed some of the differences between the good CBD oils and the sub-par ones, you know more about CBD's activity in the body, and you can have more informed discussions with your friends about its legal status and some of the differences between hemp and marijuana.

Because of the sheer number of healing benefits and uses, it's sometimes difficult to peg CBD. Since I started writing this book, I've had so many people ask me, "So, is CBD a drug, a supplement, or an herb? Is it meant to be taken daily or only once in a while? Is it for specific conditions or general wellness?" I think the answer to all of these questions is "All of the above," because you really can think about CBD in quite a few different ways—and all of them make sense.

For starters, you can think of CBD as a targeted therapeutic agent. This would apply to people using it for severe and rare conditions like seizure disorders. Next, you can think of CBD as a new way to fight an extremely wide range of inflammatory diseases (like rheumatoid arthritis, multiple sclerosis, lupus, psoriasis—the list goes on) with fewer side effects than the existing medications. We'll be seeing a lot more research on how this will work in the future. Lastly, you can think of CBD as a daily dose of anti-inflammatory and antioxidant wellness that can be incorporated into food, drink, or a beauty routine. In this way, CBD feels more like turmeric, activated charcoal, or vitamin D.

So how does one make sense of all this? I mean, can a plant really be all these things at once? Well, it's important to know that scientists have been using plants in this way for a long time. In fact, about half of all existing pharmaceutical drugs are derived from natural compounds. Aspirin comes from the bark of a willow tree, and penicillin is made from a mold that grows on cantaloupe. Because of this, scientists are constantly combing the planet for the next lifesaving plant medicine, which is extremely tedious work, since they typically have to test thousands of plants before they find even one that shows true therapeutic value in a lab. What's the take-home message here? Plant medicine and Big Pharma aren't quite as disparate as we think—and nature is the ultimate chemist.

Knowing how closely linked natural remedies and pharmaceutical drugs really are—and how desperately scientists are scouring the planet for the next great plant medicine—it's a bit ironic that as a society we've been sitting on the great discovery that CBD and cannabis have so many healing properties. It's pretty tragic that we've known about the therapeutic properties of CBD for decades but allowed stigma and politics to prevent us from taking it seriously as a medicine. You could even go so far as to say that if we discovered cannabis for the first time tomorrow, it would change the face of medicine and be praised as a miracle plant by doctors and pharmaceutical companies and politicians alike. And though it's great that there are some clinical trials being conducted now, we have to ask the question: Why isn't there more research on CBD?

The answer to this question is actually pretty simple: Studying CBD in the United States is complicated. For starters, just to be able to conduct research on a federally classified Schedule 1 drug, researchers have to get a license from the Drug Enforcement Administration and approval from the Food and Drug Administration and the National Institute of Drug Abuse (NIDA). Getting approval from three federal agencies means a lot of confusing paperwork, and the process is anything but streamlined. To paint a picture, imagine that to obtain a driver's license you had to get approved by the Internal Revenue Service, the United States Post Office, *and* the Department of Motor Vehicles, all with different requirements, long lines, and reams of paperwork—none of which could be processed electronically. In theory, all this red tape makes sense for harmful substances—you don't want just anyone approved to have a laboratory full of drugs (especially since other Schedule 1 substances include heroin and LSD)—but in reality, it prevents us from learning anything of value about CBD.

Ironically, it might actually be easier to study drugs like LSD than to study cannabis and its derivatives. This is because scientists studying LSD and other controlled substances can get it from private manufacturers who are qualified to produce and dispense it, but scientists studying cannabis can get their material only from NIDA—which gets it only from the University of Mississippi. (Yes, I did say Mississippi.) It might feel like I'm pulling your leg, but I'm not; shockingly, since 1968, UM has been the lone NIDA-approved legal marijuana grower and distributor in the country.

This is definitely strange, but it's not the end of the world. That is, until you learn that this Mississippi cannabis is famously low quality. This means that even if researchers from California (where high-quality therapeutic cannabis is being produced, is grown under a state license, and is tested at a state lab) want to study one of the benefits of cannabis, they still have to use the subpar plants supplied by NIDA to conduct legitimate research.

All of this sounds frustrating, but it's even worse when you apply it to a real-life scenario. In an interview with *Rolling Stone*, a researcher in California named Dr. Sue Sisley said that it took seven years to get approval from the federal government to study the effects of marijuana on veterans with PTSD. She then had to wait twenty months to get NIDA-sourced cannabis, and when she received the samples, she discovered that they didn't meet the potency requirements for her study. Oh, and they were also contaminated with mold. The scary part? Sisley and her colleagues were actually the first researchers to conduct secondary testing of the NIDA cannabis, which means that the cannabis used in research in the United States has likely never been checked for quality, which could majorly skew data and results.

In 2011, the Drug Enforcement Administration did change some rules to allow other producers to supply cannabis for research purposes. They received over twenty applications from growers who would likely be able to supply safer, higher quality, and more potent material to use in research, and just needed final approval from the Justice Department. They have yet to receive it.

Clearly, there's a lot of room for improvement, and I could talk about it all day, but there is just one important point to take home, and that is the fact that despite all of the restrictions against CBD research, there are hundreds of thousands of Americans using cannabis and CBD to help manage their illnesses. Some people are getting it from a high-end dispensary or from hemp-based sources and others are getting it from the 7-Eleven parking lot, but people are using it, and we owe it to them to study it to make sure it's safe.

If you've gotten to this section of the book, I hope that you feel like you have learned more about CBD. And whether you're a veteran CBD user, a newbie, or still a complete skeptic, I want to thank you for taking this journey with me. Admittedly, there's still a lot to learn about CBD, but research has already suggested that CBD may have immune-system-regulating, anti-inflammatory, antianxiety, antidepressant, anti-seizure, neuroprotective, and pain-relieving properties in a world that is desperate for more treatment options for these very complaints. But with so many obstacles standing between us and high-quality research on CBD, we're left only with opinions, biases, and beliefs—which won't lead us anywhere except to years and years of arguing and debate. The millions of people suffering from these conditions every single day deserve better; they deserve facts and the truth. Two things that are more important now than ever before.

RESOURCES

Alhamoruni, A., K. L. Wright, M. Larvin, and S. E. O'Sullivan. "Cannabinoids Mediate Opposing Effects on Inflammation-Induced Intestinal Permeability." *British Journal of Pharmacology* 165, no. 8 (April 2012): 2598–2610. https://doi.org/10.1111/j.1476-5381.2011.01589.x.

Alvarez, Francisco J., Hector Lafuente, M. Carmen Rey-Santano, Victoria E. Mielgo, Elena Gastiasoro, Miguel Rueda, Roger G. Pertwee, Ana I. Castillo, Julián Romero, and José Martínez-Orgado. "Neuroprotective Effects of the Nonpsychoactive Cannabinoid Cannabidiol in Hypoxic-Ischemic Newborn Piglets." *Pediatric Research* 64, no. 6 (December 2008): 653–58. https://doi.org/10.1203/PDR.0b013e318186e5dd.

Armstrong, Jane L., David S. Hill, Christopher S. McKee, Sonia Hernandez-Tiedra, Mar Lorente, Israel Lopez-Valero, Maria Eleni Anagnostou, et al. "Exploiting Cannabinoid-Induced Cytotoxic Autophagy to Drive Melanoma Cell Death." *The Journal of Investigative Dermatology* 135, no. 6 (June 2015): 1629–37. https://doi.org/10.1038/jid.2015.45.

Aso, Ester, Alexandre Sánchez-Pla, Esteban Vegas-Lozano, Rafael Maldonado, and Isidro Ferrer. "Cannabis-Based Medicine Reduces Multiple Pathological Processes in AßPP/PS1 Mice." *Journal of Alzheimer's Disease* 43, no. 3 (2015): 977–91. https://doi.org/10.3233/JAD-141014.

Atakan, Zerrin. "Cannabis, a Complex Plant: Different Compounds and Different Effects on Individuals." *Therapeutic Advances in Psychopharmacology* 2, no. 6 (December 2012): 241–54. https://doi.org/10.1177/2045125312457586.

Bachhuber, Marcus A., Brendan Saloner, Chinazo O. Cunningham, and Colleen L. Barry. "Medical Cannabis Laws and Opioid Analgesic Overdose Mortality in the United States, 1999-2010." *JAMA Internal Medicine* 174, no. 10 (October 1, 2014): 1668–73. https://doi.org/10.1001/jamainternmed.2014.4005.

Bilkei-Gorzo, Andras, Onder Albayram, Astrid Draffehn, Kerstin Michel, Anastasia Piyanova, Hannah Oppenheimer, Mona Dvir-Ginzberg, et al. "A Chronic Low Dose of Δ9-Tetrahydrocannabinol (THC) Restores Cognitive Function in Old Mice." *Nature Medicine* 23, no. 6 (June 2017): 782–87. https://doi.org/10.1038/nm.4311.

Bischoff, Stephan C., Giovanni Barbara, Wim Buurman, Theo Ockhuizen, Jörg-Dieter Schulzke, Matteo Serino, Herbert Tilg, Alastair Watson, and Jerry M Wells. "Intestinal Permeability—A New Target for Disease Prevention and Therapy." *BMC Gastroenterology* 14 (November 18, 2014). https://doi.org/10.1186/s12876-014-0189-7.

Blessing, Esther M., Maria M. Steenkamp, Jorge Manzanares, and Charles R. Marmar. "Cannabidiol as a Potential Treatment for Anxiety Disorders." *Neurotherapeutics* 12, no. 4 (October 2015): 825–36. https://doi.org/10.1007/s13311-015-0387-1.

Blüher, Matthias, Stefan Engeli, Nora Klöting, Janin Berndt, Mathias Fasshauer, Sándor Bátkai, Pál Pacher, Michael R. Schön, Jens Jordan, and Michael Stumvoll. "Dysregulation of the Peripheral and Adipose Tissue Endocannabinoid System in Human Abdominal Obesity." *Diabetes* 55, no. 11 (November 2006): 3053–60. https://doi.org/10.2337/db06-0812.

Booz, George W. "Cannabidiol as an Emergent Therapeutic Strategy for Lessening the Impact of Inflammation on Oxidative Stress." *Free Radical Biology & Medicine* 51, no. 5 (September 1, 2011): 1054–61. https://doi.org/10.1016/j.freeradbiomed.2011.01.007.

"Cannabidiol as a Different Type of an Antipsychotic: Drug Delivery and Interaction Study—Tabular View—ClinicalTrials.gov." Accessed May 26, 2018. https://clinicaltrials.gov/ct2/show/record/NCT02051387.

"Cannabidiol as a Treatment for AUD Comorbid With PTSD—Full Text View—ClinicalTrials.gov." Accessed May 26, 2018. https://clinicaltrials.gov/ct2/show/NCT03248167.

"Cannabidiol for Inflammatory Bowel Disease—No Study Results Posted—ClinicalTrials.gov." Accessed May 26, 2018. https://clinicaltrials.gov/ct2/show/results/NCT01037322.

Chagas, Marcos Hortes N., Antonio W. Zuardi, Vitor Tumas, Márcio Alexandre Pena-Pereira, Emmanuelle T. Sobreira, Mateus M. Bergamaschi, Antonio Carlos dos Santos, Antonio Lucio Teixeira, Jaime E. C. Hallak, and José Alexandre S. Crippa. "Effects of Cannabidiol in the Treatment of Patients with Parkinson's Disease: An Exploratory Double-Blind Trial." *Journal of Psychopharmacology (Oxford, England)* 28, no. 11 (November 2014): 1088–98. https://doi.org/10.1177/0269881114550355.

Chakrabarti, Bhismadev, Antonio Persico, Natalia Battista, and Mauro Macca-rrone. "Endocannabinoid Signaling in Autism." *Neurotherapeutics* 12, no. 4 (October 1, 2015): 837–47. https://doi.org/10.1007/s13311-015-0371-9.

CNN, By Saundra Young. "Marijuana Stops Child's Severe Seizures." CNN. Accessed November 25, 2017. http://www.cnn.com/2013/08/07/health/charlotte-child-medical-marijuana/index.html.

Costa, Barbara, Gabriella Giagnoni, Chiara Franke, Anna Elisa Trovato, and Mariapia Colleoni. "Vanilloid TRPV1 Receptor Mediates the Antihyperalgesic Effect of the Nonpsychoactive Cannabinoid, Cannabidiol, in a Rat Model of Acute Inflammation." *British Journal of Pharmacology* 143, no. 2 (September 2004): 247–50. https://doi.org/10.1038/sj.bjp.0705920.

Croxford, J. Ludovic. "Therapeutic Potential of Cannabinoids in CNS Disease." *CNS Drugs* 17, no. 3 (2003): 179–202.

Cunha, J. M., E. A. Carlini, A. E. Pereira, O. L. Ramos, C. Pimentel, R. Gagliardi, W. L. Sanvito, N. Lander, and R. Mechoulam. "Chronic Administration of Cannabidiol to Healthy Volunteers and Epileptic Patients." *Pharmacology* 21, no. 3 (1980): 175–85. https://doi.org/10.1159/000137430.

Dhital, Saphala, John V. Stokes, Nogi Park, Keun-Seok Seo, and Barbara L. F. Kaplan. "Cannabidiol (CBD) Induces Functional Tregs in Response to Low-Level T Cell Activation." *Cellular Immunology* 312 (February 2017): 25–34. https://doi.org/10.1016/j.cellimm.2016.11.006.

Edwards, Tanya. "Inflammation, Pain, and Chronic Disease: An Integrative Approach to Treatment and Prevention." *Alternative Therapies in Health and Medicine* 11, no. 6 (December 2005): 20–27; quiz 28, 75.

"The Effect of CanChew® Cannabidiol (CBD) Containing Chewing Gum on Irritable Bowel Syndrome—Full Text View—ClinicalTrials.gov." Accessed May 26, 2018. https://clinicaltrials.gov/ct2/show/NCT03003260.

Gable, Robert. "The Toxicity of Recreational Drugs." *American Scientist* 94, no. 3 (June 2006): 206. doi:10.1511/2006.3.206.

Gertsch, Jürg, Roger G Pertwee, and Vincenzo Di Marzo. "Phytocannabinoids beyond the Cannabis Plant—Do They Exist?" *British Journal of Pharmacology* 160, no. 3 (June 2010): 523–29. https://doi.org/10.1111/j.1476-5381.2010.00745.x.

Gururajan, Anand, David A. Taylor, and Daniel T. Malone. "Cannabidiol and Clozapine Reverse MK-801-Induced Deficits in Social Interaction and Hyperactivity in Sprague-Dawley Rats." *Journal of Psychopharmacology* 26, no. 10 (October 2012): 1317–32. https://doi.org/10.1177/0269881112441865.

Hampson, A. J., M. Grimaldi, J. Axelrod, and D. Wink. "Cannabidiol and (-) Δ9-Tetrahydrocannabinol Are Neuroprotective Antioxidants." *Proceedings of the National Academy of Sciences of the United States of America* 95, no. 14 (July 7, 1998): 8268–73.

Harvard Health. "Playing with the Fire of Inflammation." Harvard Health. Accessed May 26, 2018. https://www.health.harvard.edu/staying-healthy/playing-with-the-fire-of-inflammation.

Hill, Matthew N., Linda M. Bierer, Iouri Makotkine, Julia A. Golier, Sandro Galea, Bruce S. McEwen, Cecilia J. Hillard, and Rachel Yehuda. "Reductions in Circulating Endocannabinoid Levels in Individuals with Post-Traumatic Stress Disorder Following Exposure to the World Trade Center Attacks." *Psychoneuroendocrinology* 38, no. 12 (December 2013). https://doi.org/10.1016/j.psyneuen.2013.08.004.

Hill, Matthew N., Gregory E. Miller, Erica J. Carrier, Boris B. Gorzalka, and Cecilia J. Hillard. "Circulating Endocannabinoids and N-Acyl Ethanolamines Are Differentially Regulated in Major Depression and Following Exposure to Social Stress." *Psychoneuroendocrinology* 34, no. 8 (September 2009): 1257–62. https://doi.org/10.1016/j.psyneuen.2009.03.013.

Iseger, Tabitha A., and Matthijs G. Bossong. "A Systematic Review of the Antipsychotic Properties of Cannabidiol in Humans." *Schizophrenia Research* 162, no. 1–3 (March 2015): 153–61. https://doi.org/10.1016/j.schres.2015.01.033.

Izzo, Angelo A., Francesca Borrelli, Raffaele Capasso, Vincenzo Di Marzo, and Raphael Mechoulam. "Non-Psychotropic Plant Cannabinoids: New Therapeutic Opportunities from an Ancient Herb." *Trends in Pharmacological Sciences* 30, no. 10 (October 2009): 515–27. https://doi.org/10.1016/j.tips.2009.07.006.

Kogan, Natalya M., and Raphael Mechoulam. "Cannabinoids in Health and Disease." *Dialogues in Clinical Neuroscience* 9, no. 4 (December 2007): 413–30.

———. "The Chemistry of Endocannabinoids." *Journal of Endocrinological Investigation* 29, no. 3 Suppl (2006): 3–14.

Lafourcade, Mathieu, Thomas Larrieu, Susana Mato, Anais Duffaud, Marja Sepers, Isabelle Matias, Veronique De Smedt-Peyrusse, et al. "Nutritional Omega-3 Deficiency Abolishes Endocannabinoid-Mediated Neuronal Functions." *Nature Neuroscience* 14, no. 3 (March 2011): 345–50. https://doi.org/10.1038/nn.2736.

Laprairie, R. B., A. M. Bagher, M. E. M. Kelly, and E. M. Denovan-Wright. "Cannabidiol Is a Negative Allosteric Modulator of the Cannabinoid CB1 Receptor." *British Journal of Pharmacology* 172, no. 20 (n.d.): 4790–4805. https://doi.org/10.1111/bph.13250.

Lee, Martin A. *Smoke Signals: A Social History of Marijuana—Medical, Recreational and Scientific.* New York: Scribner, 2013.

Libro, Rosaliana, Francesca Diomede, Domenico Scionti, Adriano Piattelli, Gianpaolo Grassi, Federica Pollastro, Placido Bramanti, Emanuela Mazzon, and Oriana Trubiani. "Cannabidiol Modulates the Expression of Alzheimer's Disease-Related Genes in Mesenchymal Stem Cells." *International Journal of Molecular Sciences* 18, no. 1 (December 23, 2016): 26. https://doi.org/10.3390/ijms18010026.

Maccarrone, M., and A. Finazzi-Agró. "The Endocannabinoid System, Anandamide and the Regulation of Mammalian Cell Apoptosis." *Cell Death and Differentiation* 10, no. 9 (September 2003): 946–55. https://doi.org/10.1038/sj.cdd.4401284.

Massi, Paola, Angelo Vaccani, Stefania Ceruti, Arianna Colombo, Maria P. Abbracchio, and Daniela Parolaro. "Antitumor Effects of Cannabidiol, a Nonpsychoactive Cannabinoid, on Human Glioma Cell Lines." *The Journal of Pharmacology and Experimental Therapeutics* 308, no. 3 (March 2004): 838–45. https://doi.org/10.1124/jpet.103.061002.

Mead, Alice. "The Legal Status of Cannabis (marijuana) and Cannabidiol (CBD) under U.S. Law." *Epilepsy & Behavior* 70, no. Pt B (2017): 288–91. https://doi.org/10.1016/j.yebeh.2016.11.021.

Mechoulam, R., and Y. Shvo. "Hashish. I. The Structure of Cannabidiol." *Tetrahedron* 19, no. 12 (1963): 2073–78.

Mikos, Robert A. *Marijuana Law, Policy, and Authority.* New York: Wolters Kluwer, 2017.

Morales, Paula, and Patricia H. Reggio. "An Update on Non-CB1, Non-CB2 Cannabinoid Related G-Protein-Coupled Receptors." *Cannabis and Cannabinoid Research* 2, no. 1 (October 1, 2017): 265–73. https://doi.org/10.1089/can.2017.0036.

Mounessa, Jessica S., Julia A. Siegel, Cory A. Dunnick, and Robert P. Dellavalle. "The Role of Cannabinoids in Dermatology." *Journal of the American Academy of Dermatology* 77, no. 1 (2017): 188–90. https://doi.org/10.1016/j.jaad.2017.02.056.

Muller, Tania, Laurent Demizieux, Stéphanie Troy-Fioramonti, Joseph Gresti, Jean-Paul Pais de Barros, Hélène Berger, Bruno Vergès, and Pascal Degrace. "Overactivation of the Endocannabinoid System Alters the Antilipolytic Action of Insulin in Mouse Adipose Tissue." *American Journal of Physiology, Endocrinology and Metabolism* 313, no. 1 (01 2017): E26–36. https://doi.org/10.1152/ajpendo.00374.2016.

Murillo-Rodríguez, Eric, Diana Millán-Aldaco, Marcela Palomero-Rivero, Raphael Mechoulam, and René Drucker-Colín. "The Nonpsychoactive Cannabis Constituent Cannabidiol Is a Wake-Inducing Agent." *Behavioral Neuroscience* 122, no. 6 (December 2008): 1378–82. https://doi.org/10.1037/a0013278.

———. "Effects on sleep and dopamine levels of microdialysis perfusion of cannabidiol into the lateral hypothalamus of rats." *Life Sciences* 88, no. 11–12 (March 14, 2011): 504–11.

Nagarkatti, Prakash, Rupal Pandey, Sadiye Amcaoglu Rieder, Venkatesh L Hegde, and Mitzi Nagarkatti. "Cannabinoids as Novel Anti-Inflammatory Drugs." *Future Medicinal Chemistry* 1, no. 7 (October 2009): 1333–49. https://doi.org/10.4155/fmc.09.93.

Neumeister, Alexander. "The Endocannabinoid System Provides an Avenue for Evidence-Based Treatment Development for PTSD." *Depression and Anxiety* 30, no. 2 (n.d.): 93–96. https://doi.org/10.1002/da.22031.

O'Connell, Brooke K., David Gloss, and Orrin Devinsky. "Cannabinoids in Treatment-Resistant Epilepsy: A Review." *Epilepsy & Behavior* 70, no. Pt B (2017): 341–48. https://doi.org/10.1016/j.yebeh.2016.11.012.

Oláh, Attila, Balázs I. Tóth, István Borbíró, Koji Sugawara, Attila G. Szöllõsi, Gabriella Czifra, Balázs Pál, et al. "Cannabidiol Exerts Sebostatic and Antiinflammatory Effects on Human Sebocytes." *The Journal of Clinical Investigation* 124, no. 9 (September 2014): 3713–24. https://doi.org/10.1172/JCI64628.

Pacher, Pál, Sándor Bátkai, and George Kunos. "The Endocannabinoid System as an Emerging Target of Pharmacotherapy." *Pharmacological Reviews* 58, no. 3 (September 2006): 389–462. https://doi.org/10.1124/pr.58.3.2.

Pertwee, Roger G. "Cannabinoid Pharmacology: The First 66 Years." *British Journal of Pharmacology* 147, no. Suppl 1 (January 2006): S163–71. https://doi.org/10.1038/sj.bjp.0706406.

Pham-Huy, Lien Ai, Hua He, and Chuong Pham-Huy. "Free Radicals, Antioxidants in Disease and Health." *International Journal of Biomedical Science* 4, no. 2 (June 2008): 89–96.

Prud'homme, Mélissa, Romulus Cata, and Didier Jutras-Aswad. "Cannabidiol as an Intervention for Addictive Behaviors: A Systematic Review of the Evidence." *Substance Abuse: Research and Treatment* 9 (May 21, 2015): 33–38. https://doi.org/10.4137/SART.S25081.

Reiman, Amanda, Mark Welty, and Perry Solomon. "Cannabis as a Substitute for Opioid-Based Pain Medication: Patient Self-Report." *Cannabis and Cannabinoid Research* 2, no. 1 (June 1, 2017): 160–66. https://doi.org/10.1089/can.2017.0012.

Russo, Ethan B. "Taming THC: Potential Cannabis Synergy and Phytocannabinoid-Terpenoid Entourage Effects." *British Journal of Pharmacology* 163, no. 7 (August 2011): 1344–64. https://doi.org/10.1111/j.1476-5381.2011.01238.x.

Russo, Ethan B., Andrea Burnett, Brian Hall, and Keith K. Parker. "Agonistic Properties of Cannabidiol at 5-HT1a Receptors." *Neurochemical Research* 30, no. 8 (August 2005): 1037–43. https://doi.org/10.1007/s11064-005-6978-1.

Sarchielli, Paola, Luigi Alberto Pini, Francesca Coppola, Cristiana Rossi, Antonio Baldi, Maria Luisa Mancini, and Paolo Calabresi. "Endocannabinoids in Chronic Migraine: CSF Findings Suggest a System Failure." *Neuropsychopharmacology* 32, no. 6 (June 2007): 1384–90. https://doi.org/10.1038/sj.npp.1301246.

Shannon, Scott, and Janet Opila-Lehman. "Cannabidiol Oil for Decreasing Addictive Use of Marijuana: A Case Report." *Integrative Medicine* 14, no. 6 (December 2015): 31–35.

Smith, Steele Clarke, and Mark S. Wagner. "Clinical Endocannabinoid Deficiency (CECD) Revisited: Can This Concept Explain the Therapeutic Benefits of Cannabis in Migraine, Fibromyalgia, Irritable Bowel Syndrome and Other Treatment-Resistant Conditions?" *Neuro Endocrinology Letters* 35, no. 3 (2014): 198–201.

"Study of Four Different Potencies of Smoked Marijuana in 76 Veterans With PTSD—Full Text View—ClinicalTrials.gov." Accessed May 26, 2018. https://clinicaltrials.gov/ct2/show/NCT02759185.

"Study to Test the Safety and Efficacy of Cannabidiol as a Treatment Intervention for Opioid Relapse—Full Text View—ClinicalTrials.gov." Accessed May 26, 2018. https://clinicaltrials.gov/ct2/show/NCT01311778.

Thiele, Elizabeth A., Eric D. Marsh, Jacqueline A. French, Maria Mazurkiewicz-Beldzinska, Selim R. Benbadis, Charuta Joshi, Paul D. Lyons, et al. "Cannabidiol in Patients with Seizures Associated with Lennox-Gastaut Syndrome (GWPCARE4): A Randomised, Double-Blind, Placebo-Controlled Phase 3 Trial." *The Lancet* 391, no. 10125 (March 17, 2018): 1085–96. https://doi.org/10.1016/S0140-6736(18)30136-3.

Tovar, Juan Camilo Maldonado. "Meet the 'Father of Cannabis,' the Man Who Discovered Why Weed Makes You High." *Vice*, February 19, 2016. www.vice.com/en_us/article/mvxde4/raphael-mechulam-father-cannabis -discover-thc.

"U of U Health." healthcare.utah.edu. Accessed May 26, 2018. https://health care.utah.edu/.

Vogt, Nicholas M., Robert L. Kerby, Kimberly A. Dill-McFarland, Sandra J. Harding, Andrew P. Merluzzi, Sterling C. Johnson, Cynthia M. Carlsson, et al. "Gut Microbiome Alterations in Alzheimer's Disease." *Scientific Reports* 7, no. 1 (October 19, 2017): 13537. https://doi.org/10.1038/s41598-017-13601-y.

Welty, Timothy E., Adrienne Luebke, and Barry E. Gidal. "Cannabidiol: Promise and Pitfalls." *Epilepsy Currents* 14, no. 5 (2014): 250–52. https:// doi.org/10.5698/1535-7597-14.5.250.

Wilkinson, Jonathan D., and Elizabeth M. Williamson. "Cannabinoids Inhibit Human Keratinocyte Proliferation through a Non-CB1/CB2 Mechanism and Have a Potential Therapeutic Value in the Treatment of Psoriasis." *Journal of Dermatological Science* 45, no. 2 (February 1, 2007): 87–92. https:// doi.org/10.1016/j.jdermsci.2006.10.009.

Witkamp, Renger, and Jocelijn Meijerink. "The Endocannabinoid System: An Emerging Key Player in Inflammation." *Current Opinion in Clinical Nutrition and Metabolic Care* 17, no. 2 (March 2014): 130–38. https://doi.org/10.1097/ MCO.0000000000000027.

ACKNOWLEDGMENTS

Thank you to my mom, for learning how to use Google Docs to help with my manuscript. Thank you for being there for me every single step of the way—I'd be nowhere if it wasn't for you!

Thank you to my dad, for having great ideas (even if I resist them at first) and for giving me a brain that likes to think outside the box. You've always forged your own path and it makes me want to do the same!

Thank you to my amazing agent, Anna: your positivity and confidence in me propelled me through this process.

Thank you to my wonderful editor, Róisín. It's been a pleasure to create this book with you and I'm so excited that together, we get to share CBD oil with the world!

Thank you to Dr. Lester, for your words of encouragement and for writing such a wonderful foreword. Your hard work sharing functional medicine with others means so much!

To all the doctors, researchers, business owners, and cannabis growers who I interviewed for this book. Thank you for sharing your hard-earned knowledge with me. I wouldn't know anything about CBD if it wasn't for you!

Thank you to Miachel Breton, for your wonderful photography, creative direction, and for taking me on my first trip to BLICK.

Thank you to my sister Hannah, for being a strong, confident, smart, badass woman that I've always looked up to. I'm so glad we share the same love of rosé and terrible teen movies.

Thank you to my bestie, Hannah Montague, who came to NYC and ended up working an 11-hour day without a single complaint. Thank you for always, always laughing with me and for keeping me sane!

A big thank you to Liz Moody, you have saved my ass more than once. You really are the best kind of Leo.

Thank you to my Uncle Jim, for the words of encouragement, all the Sunday night dinners, and sharing your thoughts and wisdom with me. I'm so lucky!

Thank you to Bobbitt, Lauren, Elle, Krysten, and Jenna, for being the world's best resources, LA tour guides, hand models, and friends, too.

Thank you to mindbodygreen, especially the editorial team, for giving me the opportunity to share my deep love of health and wellness with such an amazing community of like-minded people.

INDEX

Note: Page references in *italics* indicate photographs.

ABOUT THE AUTHOR

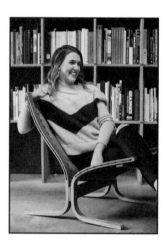

Gretchen Lidicker is the health editor for mindbodygreen.com—one of the world's top health and wellness websites—and has worked on the academic and clinical side of integrative medicine for many years. She has a masters degree in physiology and biophysics with a concentration on complementary and alternative medicine from Georgetown University. Originally from Sedona, Arizona, where she was first exposed to natural medicine, Lidicker lives in New York City.